On the Normalization
of Organized Brutalities

Dennis Firkus

On the Normalization
of Organized Brutalities

An Organizational Sociological
Analysis of the Euthanasia Institution
Hadamar

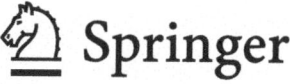 Springer

Dennis Firkus
Bielefeld, Germany

ISBN 978-3-658-41514-3   ISBN 978-3-658-41515-0   (eBook)
https://doi.org/10.1007/978-3-658-41515-0

"Euthanasia" is omitted, and what remains is the mass killing of such people who, from the point of view of purely material usefulness or for racial or even political reasons, were not desired by the political and state leadership of the time. It was not "euthanasia" in the narrower or broader sense, not the carrying out of a task borne by a sense of ethical responsibility and serious science, but a planned mass extermination of whole groups of undesirable life, carried out as brutally as it was without restraint.[1]

I was repeatedly told by the authorities in charge of me that the elimination of the incurably ill was also a matter

---

[1] Excerpt from the final verdict in the "Hadamar trial", in which a large number of members of the former euthanasia institution were tried (HHStA/b, p. 12).

promoted by the Reich and that I was serving a merciful cause in this matter. […] If I am now reproached for having actively participated in the elimination of the sick, I must confirm this. I realize today that at that time, blindly following obedience, I participated in the killing of the sick.[2]

---

[2] Statement of the nurse Paul Reuter in an interview, some decades after the end of the murders in Hadamar (quoted from Kneuker and Steglich 1985, p. 29).

Contents

Beyond Simple Explanations: An Introduction to Euthanasia

Despite its comparatively short period of rule, Germany's National Socialist regime is still considered "the most genocidal the world has ever seen" (Mann 2000, p. 331). One of the many internal campaigns to which numerous population groups and ethnic groups had to expose themselves concerned the registration and murder of physically, psychologically or mentally ill or handicapped people. In the National Socialist vocabulary, the action was translated to "euthanasia", in order to suggest an easy, honourable death by mercy, which was to be granted at most to the seriously ill. Behind this staged façade which concealed or withheld the actual intentions, a National Socialist extermination program emerged, taking into account extremely interpreted utilitarian considerations that resulted in approximately 200,000 human victims (Aly 2013, p. 9; Sandner 2003, p. 9). An alleged medical treatment of the sick, as actually practiced by psychiatric or nursing institutions, gave way to a "medicalized killing" (Lifton 1988, p. 2), which for several years was to follow the motto "cure through extermination" – or, put differently, "killing as a therapeutic imperative" (ibid., p. 21), that, as we know today, was by no means based on the idea of granting anyone a death by mercy in the true sense (Roer and Henkel 1996b, p. 24f.).

In the face of such overwhelming and depressing evidence about these and many other atrocities under the National Socialism regime, the desire for appropriate explanations is great, but the search for them is often diffuse. Many interpretations, for instance based on binary notions of personality – good and evil, persons

---

While the remarks and historical details shared throughout the book try to be as close to reality as they can be, some pseudonyms for the people involved had to be used occasionally.

acting morally or amorally, etc. –, therefore fall back on highly simplified causal explanations and perpetrator models that can above all never be definitively proven (Welzer 2005, pp. 12, 21; similarly Firkus 2017, p. 1): It were, according to a quite common diagnosis of the events in the immediate postwar period within the scholarly subsystem, the evil, barbaric personalities with sadistic dispositions in a society already manipulated by Hitler, who were driven by anti-Semitic ideas and could finally give free rein to their hatred under the leadership of the Nazi regime (Adams and Balfour 2009, p. 36; Hilberg 1989, p. 120f.; Hoffmann 2010, p. 252; Kühl 2014a, p. 7ff.).

Interpretations that, through the personalization of events, imposed responsibilities and attributions of guilt on a few and, above all, very specific participants (Kühl 2014a, p. 7), were gratefully accepted for a long time. Not only did they have a cross-generational exculpatory and guilt-dispensing effect on large sections of society itself (see for example Kühl 2013a, c), but the reference to the concealing formula of *the past*, which was far away in time as well as factually and socially, also made it possible to maintain a certain distance from the events (Adams et al. 2006, p. 690; Adams and Balfour 2009, p. 151; Lelle 2018).[1]

While these and many other, very similar explanatory approaches have certainly served their purpose of relieving responsibility sometimes more, sometimes less well, it can be stated from a scientific perspective that such interpretations are very limited in their explanatory content and thus also quickly reach their limits in terms of argumentation: We can, for example, convincingly demonstrate through a meanwhile hardly manageable variety of available sources, that the "simple explanations" suggested are simply not empirically tenable in the case of the numerous episodes of National Socialist violence (on the methodology of "problematizing the obvious", see Abbott 2004, pp. 120, 123ff.). Above all, however, these views stand in the way of analytical perspectives that seek to highlight the social dynamics and processes that are actually relevant (Kühl 2014a, p. 7f.; Welzer 2005, p. 42; also Katz 1993, p. 21). For National Socialist euthanasia, for instance, we can state that at least a large part of the (co-)perpetrators and helpers who are the focus of

---

[1] Incidentally, in the case of illegitimate or even illegal deviations, it is not unusual to personalise responsibility for action in such a form and to personify the (supposed) evil. Organizations in particular make use of such strategies to maintain legitimacy in the event of a crisis (Ermann and Lundman 1978, p. 56; Luhmann 1995, p. 114). Accordingly, this approach can be observed not only in the explanation of major historical events, but in a variety of organizational failures in general (Culjak 2015; Kühl 2020a). While in these discourses personal and stigmatizing attributions of responsibility are the rule rather than the exception, it is precisely a merit of (organizational) sociologically sensitive studies to intervene at these points and to enable precise analytical insights far removed from personal attributions of blame (Hartz 2020, p. 204; Kühl 2020a).

this book were by no means fundamentally evil or brutal excess offenders (Klee 1986, p. 94). Rather, despite all initial astonishment, it must be acknowledged that these were largely people who, in view of their background and education, were not instructed to murder, but who nevertheless participated in the events seemingly without problem or resistance and, all in all, almost without exception, engaged in beneficial activities for the National Socialist purposes – often undoubtedly only half-heartedly, perhaps in changeable proactivity, but ultimately refraining from significant protest or resistance in the overwhelming majority of cases (Hoffmann 2010; Jütte 2011, p. 99; Roer and Henkel 1996b, p. 31f.; Sandner 2003, p. 428f.).

1.1 The Organizational Involvement of the Perpetrators and Acts: A Puzzle in Need of Explanation

Following on from these circumstances, which are only hinted at for the time being and which at first glance certainly seem strange, I would like to make a contribution to explaining the empirical puzzle outlined here in the present study with the help of an organizational sociological perspective. The central question I will address is, first and foremost, how and why individuals who were not trained as mass murderers could have been in a position to act as accessories in crime on such a large scale. This, first of all, requires explanation: despite all possible heterogeneity of the participants – may such variation lie, for example, in the respective level of indoctrination, identification with the eugenic campaign, general willingness to kill, or elsewhere –, National Socialist euthanasia seems to have been based on a planned, highly effective and rational killing process that was precisely regulated in its ultimate sequence, which in its origins not only had to be first established, but at the same time had to be maintained over a long period of time (Chap. 3). In the process, these procedures took on such a stable form that they could even be continued in a modified manner at a later point in time, when there was a change in some of the central (contextual) conditions of the action (Chaps. 5 and 6). Particularly controversial in this context is the fact that the group that is in analytical focus here (see Sect. 1.2) were, in view of their largely existing vocation as nurses, committed to a completely contrary professional ethos, but despite this were still able to implement the activities necessary for mass murder in everyday practice.

The assumption that I will plausibilize for this empirical puzzle in the course of this paper is that a significant part of its solution is to be located in a fundamental understanding of organizations. The origin of my thesis is the observation that all of the murders carried out in the context of the National Socialist euthanasia campaign cannot be traced back to the structureless work of individually acting perpetrators. Rather, it becomes clear that the events were integrated into an organizationally structured and planned process.[2] In fact, we are thus not dealing at any time with individuals who engage in anti-organizational illegal behavior driven by personal motives – individuals that, for example, enrich themselves with their deeds. This observation is particularly true for the Hadamar institution, which is the central subject of investigation in this study. Instead, a major premise of sociological research can be confirmed with regard to the internal execution and the accompanying legitimization of illegal, immoral as well as corrupt practices in organizations: that it is a matter of a whole grouping of organizational members who have been active within the framework of a certain quantitative as well as qualitative group strength, i.e. a common pro-organizational illegal behavior has been practiced (Anand et al. 2004; Brief et al. 2001; Ermann and Lundman 1978; Müthel 2017).[3] In this understanding, the acts of violence are precisely not due to those irrational paradoxes mentioned before. Instead, they are the consequence of coordinated, calculated structures and patterns of the murder institutions that were provided with these very intentions. In this context, therefore, there was no pronounced "execution tourism" (Welzer 2005, p. 133) or voyeurism, in which civilians or relatives attended or watched the killings off-duty in a recreational manner (ibid., p. 203ff.). The uniformly and jointly carried out killings, on the other hand, began, according to a very central finding, at the time when the perpetrators were called upon to do so as part of their membership, and they ended again as soon as they discarded their membership role.

The clarification of the formulated empirical puzzle is thus carried out via an explanation that places the organization at the center, because the numerous (co-) participants were apparently only able to legitimize their (co-)perpetration in one way or another precisely through their organizational integration, meaning they could not have constituted the deeds without their membership. At least, this is the train of thought to be pursued here. To put it somewhat more precisely, my assumption to be plausibilized in this regard is that the National Socialist organization

---

[2] The same observation is made in Stefan Kühl's organizational sociological study of the Holocaust (2014a, p. 22), which points out that more than 99% of the killings of Jews were carried out by members of violent state organizations. I am not able to give a percentage value in the present case, but I am also not aware of a single example in which violent non-state organizations participated in euthanasia, for example in the form of a pogrom motivated by eugenics.

[3] In the English-speaking world, a distinction is also made between the "corrupt organization" on the one hand and the "organization of corrupt individuals" on the other (Pinto et al. 2008; also Campbell and Göritz 2014, p. 291f.; further distinctions in Brief et al. 2001; Kühl 2020a, p. 69ff.). Of course, such pro-organisational behaviour does not per se exclude the possibility of personal benefits (Kühl 2020a, p. 65ff.).

employed and made available numerous functions and structures that were by no means unusual, but rather typical of organizations (Luhmann 1995; see also Kühl 2014a), which the members could make use of in order to institutionalize their (co-)perpetration and rationalize all physical, social, or moral blemishes simultaneously (Anand et al. 2004; Ashforth and Kreiner 1999; Kreiner et al. 2006). Meanwhile, the organisational framing of the acts served as a desolidarising, demoralising as well as responsibility-relieving mechanism towards the victims (Balcke 2001; further also Adams and Balfour 2009, p. 4; Adams 2011, p. 277). In this way, the actions of the staff were *normalized* in an extraordinary way (Ashforth and Anand 2003), which led to members characterising the acts as indifferent – their performance thus conforming to legitimate organisational expectations of action. The fact that these behaviours could be maintained in a similar or continued in a modified way later on, although central features of the processes had changed in the meantime – including the change from the once relatively anonymous method of killing to a much more direct, individual method –, was primarily due to the fact that the killings were carried out on the basis of remembered knowledge structures or interpretations on the one hand and the consideration of former interactional and/or learning experiences of the actors on the other. Crucially, the activities in this second phase of the euthanasia program could be incorporated or subordinated into previous customary behaviours and expectations that were already normalized at the time (Gioia 1992; Gioia and Poole 1984; further Ashforth and Fried 1988).

The aim of this work is to elaborate these patterns and structures theoretically and at the same time to record and present them in their empirical manifestations. The focus lies on the question of how a large number of people, in the context of their role as a member of an organization, could participate in a mass murder for which they were in no way prepared, let alone trained. To this end, the following section will first discuss some methodological classifications as well as the necessary restrictions to be placed on the contribution (Sect. 1.2). After a contextualization of the first gas murder phase of the eugenic campaign (Sect. 1.3), a theoretical chapter follows, which will introduce the analytical foundation of this monograph (Chap. 2). With the help of some central premises of systems-theoretical organizational research, the concepts of membership, formal expectations (Sect. 2.1) and a reinterpretation of the indifference zone approach will follow (Sect. 2.2). In the third chapter, the actual analysis of the first murder phase will begin, in which the willingness and obedience of the grouping studied here – the "foot soldiers of euthanasia" (for this, Sect. 1.2) – as well as the accompanying "normalization" of the acts (Chap. 2) are shown. This is done on the basis of the three pillars of normalization, beginning with the "institutionalization" of the killings (Sect. 3.1). This is followed by their "rationalization" (Sect. 3.2), which I will show on the basis of the (supposed) legality of the acts (Sect. 3.2.1), their moral or ethical recalibration (Sect. 3.2.2), the accompanying denial of responsibility (Sect. 3.2.3), of victims (Sect. 3.2.4) as well as the general denial of any harm done by the personnel (Sect. 3.2.5), the supposedly higher expediency of the acts (Sect. 3.2.6) and, lastly, the euphemistic vocabulary underlying many episodes of the operation (Sect. 3.2.7). The "socialization" of mainly new members into the offences completes the analytical three-step (Sect. 3.3). The chapter ends with a conclusion of the analysis, in which some critical objections are made with regard to the chosen approach (Sect. 3.4).

The fourth chapter addresses the ensuing change in the historical context: after the killings of the sick were briefly interrupted (Chap. 4), the personnel who had been involved in the previous action were entrusted with other tasks (Sect. 4.1). At the same time, however, the demonstrative halt to the campaign was not the end of National Socialist euthanasia (Sect. 4.2). In the second phase, Hadamar in particular was a killing facility introduced comparatively late and under special conditions, which in this respect requires its own, separate considerations with regard to the question(s) of when, how and why the institution was reopened (Chap. 5). The following sixth chapter deals with the killings and some of the peculiarities and patterns that should be emphasized in connection with the internal killing procedure at the asylum from August 1942 onwards (Chap. 6). After a descriptive account of the events (Sect. 6.1), I come to the interpretation on the basis of the medical primacy of the killings (Sect. 6.1.1), the hierarchization of patients (especially within the institution) (Sect. 6.1.2), the personnel continuities (Sect. 6.1.3), the diffusion or delegation of responsibility (Sect. 6.1.4), the repetitive cycle of killings (Sect. 6.1.5) as well as the lack of exit options for the staff (Sect. 6.1.6), that the more individual or personal drug murders of the second phase could be successfully implemented mainly due to memorized knowledge structures or interpretations and continued (interactional) experiences (Sect. 6.2). The conclusion, in which the results are recapitulated and classified (Chap. 7), is followed by some future research perspectives offered by the previous remarks, which are mainly due to the "analytical generality" of the elaborated theses (Sect. 7.1). The conclusion deals with the convictions and the consciousness of guilt of the staff (Sect. 7.2).

1.2   Methods, Sources and Obstacles of (Organizational) Sociological Euthanasia Research

For a long time, and especially in the first years or decades after the end of the Nazi regime, sociology distinguished itself by an extraordinary lack of interest in the study of National Socialist conditions (see, for example, Borggräfe and Schnitzler 2014; Christ 2011; Dahrendorf 1989; Soeffner 2014). Continuations of this collective sociological silence can sometimes be traced into the recent past (exemplified by Kühl 2013a), although a contrary trend and the accompanying dissolution of sociology's ambivalent relationship to research on National Socialism can finally be observed (Becker 2014a, b; a compact overview of the history of the discipline and its perspectives on the subject is provided by Christ 2011; Borggräfe and Schnitzler 2014).[4]

That this phase of interdisciplinary silence was additionally accompanied by a long-running debate about the sense and nonsense of a sociological perspective on episodes of National Socialism is astonishing, to say the least: sociology is a scholarly discipline that recognizes studies of gossip (Bergmann 1987), practices of amateur pornography (Lewandowski 2019), or barbecues (Pütz and Meier zu Verl 2014) as legitimate objects of inquiry (similarly in Kühl 2013a, p. 5). Meanwhile, since the "Third Reich" has been exoticized or marginalized in parts of sociology as a phenomenon beyond any normality (Baumann 1992, p. 33; Christ and Suderland 2014, p. 21; Dahrendorf 1989, pp. 671), meaning that it would allegedly lie outside the discipline's proper purview (Christ 2014, p. 357; Katz 1982, p. 511f.; Kühl 2013a, p. 4f.), it is worth pointing out two very central criteria that make a sociological examination of euthanasia or National Socialism in general exceedingly desirable: First, even an intradisciplinary labeling of the mass killings towards the pathological will not change the fact that they are still social phenomena, which are commonly the object of study in sociology (Kühl 2013a, pp. 5, 11, 2013b, p. 2ff.). Beyond this, however, the insights gained in National Socialist studies can undoubtedly be put into perspective and integrated into a more comprehensive theory or research agenda. In the present contribution, this is, to name a

---

[4]Comparatively high prominence was achieved, for example, by studies on the Holocaust, especially the Police Battalion 101 (Kühl 2014a, 2018, 2019a, b; Hoebel 2014; see also the anthology by Gruber and Kühl 2015). Following on from this, Sandkuehler's recent work (2020) on some non-German perpetrator groups of the Holocaust should also be highlighted. Sociological research on concentration camps is certainly also to be mentioned (e.g. Suderland 2014; Hauffe 2013).

potential example, the organizational sociological research on illegal practices on the one hand, their maintenance and stabilization on the other.

The touchstone of an sociological study of National Socialist issues lies primarily in the question of whether the project can offer a plausible perspective that goes beyond the usual (for example, historical or political science) approaches (Kühl 2014a, p. 327ff.). Although the claim in the present case cannot be to provide an all-encompassing explanation of the eugenic campaign, the opposite is also true: an overall analytical account of such a social phenomenon (which has so far been lacking anyways) remains incomplete without a fundamental understanding of organizational structures (ibid., p. 35) – and it is precisely at this point where the added value of such a project is to be located.

For the treatment of the "organized brutalities" (Kühl 2005, p. 105) thematized in this book, I will use the former "Landesheil- und Pflegeanstalt" (LHA) Hadamar as a central example to illustrate the implementation of an organized mass murder. Although my research concern is inspired by studies with similar questions (especially Kühl 2014a; Welzer 2005), euthanasia as an object of investigation has remained quasi completely unconsidered in sociology until now.[5] The aforementioned question(s) and theses, slightly modified with regard to the topic, thus gain relevance simply in view of the obvious deficit in the sociological literature in this regard. Following this "gap-spotting" of an altogether neglected area of research (Sandberg and Alvesson 2011), I would therefore like to make an ambitious attempt to counteract the described desideratum. In this way, following the subtitle of Stefan Kühl's monograph on the Holocaust (2014a), while not founding the sociology of euthanasia, a contribution to *the* sociology of euthanasia can and should be made (Kühl 2018, 2019a, b, p. 117), with which the potentials of an organizational sociological analysis for the topic should be hinted at – at least as far as such an undertaking can be realized within the limits set here.

Due to restrictions that must necessarily be made as well as for research pragmatic decisions, the events that occurred in connection with the so-called "child euthanasia" are left unconsidered (for this, see, for example, Aly 2013, p. 109ff.; Klee 1986, p. 237ff.; Sandner 2003, p. 532ff.; furthermore, Burlon 2009). Simultaneously, restrictive measures are required with regard to the group of employees to which the following analysis and results will refer: I will focus on the technical, the office, as well as most especially the nursing staff from Hadamar and thus relate my statements to the orderlies, nurses, morticians, cemetery gardeners,

---

[5] In the course of this paper, I therefore regularly refer back to sociological research on the Holocaust, because I believe that numerous connections for a sociological study of euthanasia can be found here.

as well as any other administrative staff. With a simultaneous exclusion of the institutional doctors, I therefore deal with the essential helpers of the eugenic operation. The central characteristic of this collective, which I will call the "foot soldiers of euthanasia" for the purpose of generalization and simplification, is a hierarchically low position within the killing institution(s).[6] This insight was also shared by the later court cases, which is why, for example, the active doctors were condemned as perpetrators or killers, while the other staff were portrayed as accomplices or co-perpetrators in the vast majority of cases (Bryant 2005, pp. 107ff., 134; Meusch 2006, p. 314; see also Sect. 7.2). In particular, it is this group of persons examined here who allowed the Hadamar killing facility to operate in an appropriate manner in the National Socialist sense and in many respects functioned as the executive organ of a systematic and planned mass murder. Within this framework, all members of this collective contributed with their individual actions, in a narrower or broader sense, to the success of the eugenic measures and, in their sum and interaction, to the goal of the "destruction of life unworthy of life", which had long since been determined and overriding at that time (HHStA/b, p. 27f.; see generally on this idea also Adams and Balfour 2009, pp. 40ff., 56; Katz 1993, p. 11; Zimbardo 2009, p. x).[7]

In order to be able to meet the formulated demands of the work in an appropriate manner, I use various sources. Their nature can be fundamentally concentrated on two central types of material: First, this concerns primary sources, which are all too often neglected by sociologists (on archival work as a form of empirical social research, see Benzecry et al. 2020; Luft 2020). Specifically, I use the records from two post-war trials that were conducted against numerous members of the Hadamar

---

[6] With the term "foot soldiers of euthanasia" I am paraphrasing the concept of "foot soldiers of extermination", which was used to describe non-German assistants in the Holocaust (Kühl 2013c, p. 5). The "foot soldiers of euthanasia" is meant to include the mentioned German employees, i.e. the (co-)perpetrators in the asylums. The essential characteristic of this grouping is a hierarchically low position within the murder factories in opposite to the more senior functionaries. In Hadamar, the latter includes above all the two main doctors, Dr. Gorgaß and Dr. Wahlmann, the higher-ranking state secretary or later administrative director of the Hadamar asylum, Alfons Klein, as well as the even higher-ranking state councilor and department head for asylums of the Nassau District Association, Fritz Bernotat. Bernotat in particular was of central importance for the organization and execution of the second phase of the euthanasia murders in the Nassau region, as will be described in detail later (Chaps. 5 and 6).

[7] A victim-centred perspective is not adopted here. Such an approach is not intended to be fundamentally discredited, but this monograph is about understanding the behaviour of the members of the organisation. A victim perspective contributes little to this issue (Kühl 2014a, p. 41).

cadre. In these trials, a total of about 30 members of the staff had to answer for their deeds (Lilienthal 2006b, p. 288f.).

The first elaboration dealt with the war crimes trial before an American military court in Wiesbaden between October 8 and 15, 1945 (summarized by Koessler 1953). The subject of this prosecution was the murder of approximately 400–500 Polish and Russian forced laborers suffering from tuberculosis by Hadamar staff between mid-1944 and March 1945 (Koessler 1953, pp. 736, 740; Lilienthal 2010, p. 107). Seven individuals were tried for these incidents (Birkenfeld et al. 2017, p. 11; Koessler 1953, p. 736). The killings were carried out by an injection of over-dosed drugs, common in the second phase of the murders (Kintner 1948, p. 15f.). For relevant references, I primarily use the uncommented trial records of Kintner (1948).

Secondly, between 24 February and 21 March 1947, the crimes committed by the Hadamar staff against the German victims was tried in Frankfurt am Main (HHStA, Dept. 461, No. 32061, Vol. 7).[8] The proceedings were directed against the two physicians working in Hadamar, Dr. Bodo Gorgaß and Dr. Adolf Wahlmann, as well as 23 other employees – a total of 11 nurses and orderlies, 10 office employees, and finally two more persons from the technical staff (Birkenfeld et al. 2017, p. 11). Inasmuch as my analytical interest in the course of this article is primarily in the "usual" patterns and killing procedures, and the murder of foreign forced laborers – in terms of numbers alone – was the exception rather than the rule, the Frankfurt trial is of significantly greater relevance to my study.

From a source-critical point of view, it should be noted that criminal trials as well as their transcriptions represent significant sources due to the researched and evaluated documents on which they are based (Finger et al. 2009, p. 13). At the same time, however, they are precisely for this reason characterized by a certain legal pragmatism that does not necessarily seem more relevant or true for a socio-logically grounded analysis than other information that has not been taken into account or is not perceived as important (Finger et al. 2009, pp. 10, 14f.; Keßelring 2018, p. 425; furthermore, Aly 1985a, p. 71f.). Although many of the historical events would undoubtedly have been difficult or impossible to reconstruct without the reconstructions made by the authorities (see for the present case, for example, Hinz-Wessels et al. 2005; Sandner 1999), the transformation of the events into a criminal causality always entails a selection of information, because it is precisely

---

[8] Where I refer to the course of the trial in the course of the work, I refer to the abbreviation HHStA/a. Since the entire final judgment is available to me in a separate document and thus also has its own page number, which is independent of the course of the trial, I refer to the source HHStA/b in these cases.

the legally significant statements and events that are of primary interest to the respective authorities or investigators (Finger et al. 2009, p. 10; further Luft 2020). The sheer incorporation and subordination of experiences into the logic of judicial proceedings already leads to very specific, predefined limitations of the information consulted, since the goal of judicial proceedings is less the search for a supposedly universal (un-)truth than for a (il-)legality determined procedurally within the legal framework – that is, the "version of the truth that the court assumes to be true on the basis of its own work" (Brückweh 2009, p. 197; see also Luhmann 1983, p. 114ff.). The fact that statements or opinions can thus be presented in an at least partially distorted way is not improbable, especially from a sociological point of view (Herrmann 1987; furthermore Kühl 2014a, p. 341) – may the reason for this only be due to the difference between what is formally said and what is actually meant, intended or noted (Cicourel 1974, pp. 207, 220; Finger and Keller 2009, p. 116ff.). The reverse case, i.e. that the "originality" of any statements is manipulated by (un-)consciously made false statements, is equally conceivable (Finger and Keller 2009, p. 119; Finger et al. 2009, p. 14).

Furthermore, it should be noted that all testimonies by the staff on which this work is based were made retrospectively. With regard to the judicial proceedings, this is therefore more than 1 year after the acts (US trial) or 2 years after the end of the campaign (German trial), but at the same time approximately 7 years after the beginning of the first murders in Hadamar. Working with this type of material is not without its problems because, on the one hand, actors in such constellations may forget minor details, especially in contexts of violence, confuse them, or illustrate them in a version of events that is idealized for those involved (Collins 2011, p. 13). Second, agents who (have to) explain and justify their behaviour tend not to legitimise their activities with their supposedly "true" intentions. Such justifications are instead, according to a common sociological objection, usually strongly influenced by the respective normative framework – here primarily judicial, but in any case with legal or police connotations. In this sense, the explanations ultimately put forward would be solely representations of motives or so-called "vocabularies of motives", which are oriented towards the respective situational circumstances and accordingly do not provide information about the actual motives for action, but about those that appear to be appropriate (Gerth and Mills 1973; Kühl 2014a, pp. 75f., 78; Mills 1940; similarly Luhmann 1983, pp. 66f., 91 ff.). The retrospectively formulated representations of motives thereby offer the option of a "post-rationalization of one's own and others' actions" (Kühl 2018, 2019a, b, p. 118; see also Mann 2000, p. 333f.), with the help of which one can, to put it pointedly, deny oneself any free will in the context of legal proceedings and present oneself as a mere bearer of an organizationally imposed role within an uncontrollable existential exceptional situation (Finger et al. 2009, p. 13f.; Kühl 2014a, pp. 75ff, 237f., 2018, 2019a, b, pp. 108, 118f.; Mills 1940, p. 906).

Ultimately, the reservations discussed here cannot be completely circumvented in view of their immanent underlying character. In no way, however, should the conclusion be drawn from this that the source genre of judicial records is thus unsuitable for sociological investigation. On the contrary, a certain plausibility can be assumed for the statements of the Hadamar personnel in the present case in my view, particularly due to the short period of time between the context of origin and the context of the trials. The legal proceedings shortly after the end of the war, i.e. still before 1948, represent exceedingly valuable material for the reason that the strategic approaches of the defendants or their criminal defense counsel, which intensified steadily as time went on, were comparatively weak at that time due to a lack of experience and references in the matter.[9] To put it differently: Precisely because the judicial proceedings to which I refer in this thesis were not conducted 5, 10 or even 20 years after the offences, it is not possible to observe in many places the solidified and/or rehearsed forms that are usually to be expected in judicial proceedings. Moreover, it is evident from this that the first-mentioned problem of retrospectivity – i.e. events that are forgotten or confused – was perhaps not a factor to be ignored (see, for example, the corrective statement of the nurse Härtle, HHStA/a, p. 72), but rather a significantly smaller factor than in other National Socialist trials – one only has to think here, for example, of the large Frankfurt Auschwitz trial, which did not end until August 1965 (Finger and Keller 2009, p. 114).

In addition, confirming these assumptions, it can be seen from certain statements or forms of expression by the staff – which very obviously originated from a vocabulary that had National Socialist connotations and/or was influenced by the eugenic campaign –, that formerly valid contextual conditions persisted to a certain extent in the processes immediately after 1945: Notions that, for example, there was talk that in Hadamar were only the "final conditions" (statement Lückoff, nursing staff, HHStA/a, p. 99), that "very bad human material […] entertained themselves in their delusions" (statement Zielke, nursing staff, HHStA/a, p. 95f.), and that these people were finally "no longer fit to live at all" (statement Schirre, office

---

[9] I owe this hint to Winfried Süß, who was able to generalize this for the legal procedures of euthanasia in principle (telephone conversation of 28.07.2020; see also Ebbinghaus 2008, p. 211ff.). Insofar as this lack of strategic approach also includes possible mutual agreements among each other, the statements made and/or confirmed by several employees are also based on a comparatively high level of credibility. The same applies to cases of self-incrimination. In order to make my arguments plausible, I will therefore, as a rule, draw on several statements made by the staff in each case in the course of my analytical approach.

staff, HHStA/a, p. 146),[10] show clear indications that once institutionalized (primarily organizational) expectations and/or framings had lingered on, which at that time had not yet been and could not yet be overlaid by situationally legitimate representations of motives (for more general methodological implications regarding terminological interpretations, see Cicourel 1974, p. 204f.; also Abbott 2004, p. 69).

Of course, this does not mean that we can therefore use the material to look into a mirror of the social reality of the time. Ultimately, one must be aware, such a bias, as implied by the mentioned vocabularies of motive, can never be completely avoided – because in principle, every communicated motive can be assumed to be a (potential) vocabulary of motive in one way or another (analogously also Finger et al. 2009, p. 14). In this respect, the seemingly positivistic conviction that it is possible to penetrate to the incontrovertible truth with regard to the genuine drives of the agents is more of a pipe dream than a realistic research concern; a noble, but at the same time naïve claim to social reality. Possibly for this very reason, the search for the supposedly universal (un-)truth is not incumbent upon judicial procedures.[11] What is decisive in this context, however, is that the aspects presented contain convincing evidence to the effect that the judicial procedures used here did not have or could not have had as strong an effect on the statements of the personnel as might perhaps be expected at first glance – which is why in the case at hand a comparatively far-reaching approximation to the social reality of the circumstances can succeed.[12]

For the purpose of verifying the numerous statements and reconstructions in court, the addition of a second block of material serves to enable critical juxtapositions where necessary (Finger et al. 2009, p. 14). With the exception, of course, of the underlying theoretical framework (especially Chap. 2), this collection consists of non-sociological independent (monographs or collected works) and dependent (the respective contributions from the collected works consulted as well as essays or articles from journals) literature. In view of the broad historical background, I have selected various works for this purpose which are to be regarded as comprehensive contributions. For the general historical nature, these include, among

---

[10] For the sake of anonymity, the names of Schirre, Bacher and Lichtefellt have been changed.

[11] This also becomes clear from a system-theoretical perspective on the procedures: For example, the legal system does not operate with the binary code "true/untrue", as one might initially assume, but with "right/unright". The code "true/untrue" is instead inherent to the scientific subsystem (Brückweh 2009, p. 196; Luhmann 1987, p. 359).

[12] I would like to thank Thomas Hoebel, Eddie Hartmann and Martin Weißmann for various references.

others, the monographs by Aly (2013), Klee (1983 and especially 1986) or Faulstich (1998). With a focus on the Hadamar asylum, the anthologies by Roer and Henkel (1996a, b) and by George et al. (2006) are noteworthy. Also of great relevance is Sandner's detailed monograph (2003) on the Nassau District Association before and during National Socialism, which focuses not exclusively but in particular on the structural peculiarities of Hadamar asylum.

I supplemented this basic literature, which forms the basis of the work, with numerous other relevant writings, which I interpreted and processed using secondary analysis (especially Chroust et al. 1989; Lilienthal 2010). Of particular advantage were some already existing discussions with former members from the LHA, which could either be found in the aforementioned anthologies (e.g. Lilienthal 2006a, b; Schmidt-von Blittersdorff et al. 1996; Wettlaufer 1996) or represent separate elaborations (Kneuker and Steglich 1985). A large part of the literature used thus deals exclusively or largely with the asylum and the killing processes in Hadamar. In the analysis of the first phase of the murders, however, I will also refer to material that contains information about other sanatoria and nursing homes occasionally. This additional information is intended to contribute to the plausibility or supplementation of any points at the appropriate places and to reduce as far as possible any bottlenecks or uncertainties that would otherwise arise from the sources. Such an approach seems entirely plausible in the case of the euthanasia murder institutions, because – at least in the context of the gas murders (Chap. 3) – there were no significant differences in the procedures of the various institutions (Schmidt-von Blittersdorff et al. 1996, p. 87; see also the testimony of Pauline Kneissler, nursing staff, who worked in the Grafeneck and Hadamar institutions, Kneuker and Steglich 1985, p. 90f.; also Friedlander 1997, pp. 157f., 164ff.). From an analytical point of view, it is also advantageous that the basic argumentation of the work can be tested against a generalisation that takes place at least to a small extent (see also Sect. 7.1).[13]

The consequence of an approach that quite deliberately refers both to non-anonymised witness statements and to the locations of the events is that no level of theoretical abstraction customary to sociology can be maintained in such an investigation, which normally invokes precisely the complete secrecy of these two

---

[13] The information obtained from this material thus stems from a reinterpretation of already known or available sources, which is a typical approach of sociological studies (Cicourel 1974, p. 209; Kühl 2014a, p. 332f.; similarly Hoebel 2014, p. 444). Precisely because the processes have been elaborated in detail by historians, it is possible to connect them with sociological concepts that are sensitive to regularities and social laws (Cicourel 1974, p. 203; Gruber and Kühl 2015, p. 8; Kühl 2014a, p. 332).

aspects (Kühl 2013a, p. 3, 2014a, p. 37). I accept this circumstance because dispensing with anonymization equally means that follow-up projects can be designed much more easily, given the empirical accuracy of the data and information formulated here (Kühl 2014a, p. 37f.; further Luft 2020, p. 321). From a research pragmatic point of view, it should also be emphasised that this allows me to be very precise in the genesis of the data, its evaluation and, finally, its presentation in the further course of the work, without at the same time getting caught in an ambivalent space in between the purpose of the conciseness of the argument on the one hand and the anonymisation of the data on the other (Kühl 2020b).[14]

Before I continue with the historical sketch in the following chapter, I would like to make one last remark regarding National Socialist terminology. Undoubtedly, an ever-flourishing, at least latently effective defamation of those who were classified as inferior, marginalized, and not infrequently elevated to the status of an opponent that has to be destroyed, belonged to this vocabulary. In this context, of course, this already concerns the concept of *euthanasia* itself, which was intended to camouflage the racial ideological ideas under the guise of scientifically, ethnically, medically, sometimes even biologically justified necessities (Aly 2013, pp. 9, 19f.; Friedlander 1997, pp. 20ff.; HHStA/b, p. 8). Although a complete distancing from this is self-evident, such a work cannot refrain from retaining certain expressions for the purpose of appropriate reconstruction, conceptual precision as well as explanation. The resulting impositions on the readership (and, incidentally, on the author himself) are therefore excused for reasons of scientific objectivity.

1.3   Aktion T4: An Empirical Case Sketch of the Gas Murder Phase

After the introductory and reflexive remarks so far, I will direct my attention in this chapter to the historical context of the eugenic action. In doing so, the presentations do not claim to undertake a detailed historical reappraisal. Especially with topics of such historical relevance, a sociological investigation can quickly degenerate into

---

[14] Empirical social researchers in particular – and this of course includes organizational researchers – may find themselves forced to subject their empirical material to deliberate manipulation in the course of the necessary anonymization of their data (Kühl 2020b). In the case at hand, however, this problematic situation is clearly less significant, if only in view of the events that took place far in the past and the associated extinction of the generation(s) from the time (Kühl 2013b, 2017a). In this respect, however, Stefan Kühl's rule of thumb, "If you don't have to anonymise anything, you haven't got anything out" (2020b, p. 65), does not apply in this context.

a mere reproduction of contemporary historical events or the pure reconstruction of an already existing result, so that elaborations in such cases are more like a "self-historicization" than an investigation generating knowledge (Kühl 2017a). The classifications are therefore intended to provide the necessary background with regard to the analysis. In this respect, they are based solely on a criterion of relevance for the present study (see Abbott 2004, p. 69f.).

Generally speaking, the aim of eugenic movements is to increase or maximise the positive genetic make-up of a population on the basis of state intervention (Bryant 2005, p. 4). In terms of Nazi "racial hygiene," this was understood to mean the "destruction of life unworthy of life" (Schmuhl 2008, p. 102, 2011a, c). The first public discussions about the right and wrong of a possible euthanasia began years before its practical implementation (Klee 1986, p. 35ff.). The discourses, which were by no means a genuinely German phenomenon (see, for example, Kühl 1994; Schmuhl 2011b), already addressed at this early stage possible moral as well as legal limits to the killing of people who suffered from physical, mental and psychological disabilities or illnesses (Debus et al. 1996, p. 41ff.; Kaiser et al. 1992, p. 200f.; Klee 1986, p. 46ff.).[15]

The organization of Nazi (adult) euthanasia finally begins in 1939. In October, Adolf Hitler signs a document that dates back to the first of September, the invasion of Poland and the concomitant beginning of the war. In that letter, which later becomes known as the "euthanasia authorization," Hitler appoints Philipp Bouhler, Chief of the Führer's Chancellery and Reich Leader, and Karl Brand, his personal escort physician, as the leaders of the project (Aly 2013, p. 24f.; Klee 1983, p. 11, 1986, p. 20). Officially, it states:

> Reich Leader Bouhler and Dr. med. Brandt are charged with the responsibility of enlarging the competence of certain physicians, designated by name, so that patients

---

[15] In the National Socialist context, the concept of „life unworthy of life" first gains relevance in 1920. In this year, in connection with the poor quality of life during and after the lost war, a brochure appears with the (here translated) title: "The Permission to Destroy Life Unworthy of Life. Its Measure and Form" (Aly 2013, p. 21; Klee 1986, p. 37; see also Bryant 2005, p. 21ff.). Even in this early version, the idea of eugenically justified killing is oriented and justified by the value of the human being, here in the form of a rhetorical question intended to draw attention to the fact that the murder of certain individuals would be worthwhile: "Is there human life which has so far forfeited the character of something entitled to enjoy the protection of the law that its prolongation represents a perpetual loss of value, both for its bearer and for society as a whole?" (quoted in Bryant 2005, p. 21). At a later stage, this work was to become a theoretical basis for the murder of the sick (Kneuker and Steglich 1985, p. 10f.; Schmuhl 2011c, p. 216).

who, on the basis of human judgment, are considered incurable, can be granted mercy death after a discerning diagnosis. (quoted from Klee 1986, p. 85)

In fact, this was the only document Hitler ever signed himself in connection with the killing of the handicapped and mentally ill (statement by Heyde, former senior medical expert, HHStA/a, p. 342).[16]

In future, this letter would serve in internal circles as a legitimizing – albeit not legalizing (see Sect. 3.2.1) – basis for the measures proclaimed. The two euthanasia authorizers were thereby granted the authority to subsequently set up a program that was to systematically record and exterminate those people who, in view of physical, mental and/or psychological disabilities, no longer appeared fit for work (Klee 1986, pp. 85f., 100f.). Basically, the assessment of selected human qualities was based on an extreme rationality principle, which could be translated into a simple, but at the same time brutal cost-benefit calculation: if the value of the labour power of a person (judged to be ill) was less than the costs he or she caused for the "Volksgemeinschaft", this person lost his or her right to live (Roer and Henkel 1996a, p. 11, 1996b, p. 23f., 34f.).[17] The decisive criterion of segregation for the National Socialists was thus whether the individual was capable of productive or useful work (Klee 1983, pp. 118f., 177).

However, the organizational structures entrusted with the task were already established in the summer of 1939 (for confirmation that the campaign must undoubtedly have begun before September 1, 1939, see also the statement of Heyde, former senior medical expert, HHStA/a, p. 341). A short time later, in April 1940, the newly established Central Office (*Zentraldienststelle*) in Berlin was occupied – located at Tiergartenstraße 4, which is why the project is known today as "Aktion

---

[16] In the end, however, the chief organizer of the eugenic campaign was not the head of the chancellery Bouhler, but the department head Viktor Brack, usually identified in official documents under the pseudonym "Jennerwein" (Klee 1986, p. 130; Sandner 2003, pp. 372, 516; see also Friedlander 1997, pp. 118ff.).

[17] The exception to this were Jewish patients, who were all condemned to death, far from their possible working capacity (Schmidt-von Blittersdorff et al. 1996, p. 89). In general, a separate, quasi-special set of rules applied to the handling of Jewish patients. A "Jewish special treatment" in the first phase of euthanasia provided for the concentration of Jewish patients in selected intermediate institutions (*Zwischenanstalten*), i.e. selected only for them, including the transfer to the respective killing institutions (Hinz-Wessels et al. 2005, p. 93f.; Lilienthal 2009, p. 10; in detail in Hinz-Wessels 2002). However, Jewish patients were also transported and murdered in the conventional transports.

T4" (Debus et al. 1996, p. 49).[18] In the following weeks and months of the war, a total of six killing facilities were set up, in which patients were murdered by CO gas from January 1940 until the end of August 1941 and then incinerated or cremated immediately afterwards.[19] The processes in this so-called "gas murder phase" were made possible in all the institutions with the aid of an immense organisational effort (Hinz-Wessels et al. 2005, p. 85f.; for more details, see Sect. 3.1).

An initial assessment of the eligible patients was carried out with a written record of the later victims, which was repeated and developed over time (Schmuhl 2011c, p. 213f.). For this purpose, the bureaucratic T4 headquarters in Berlin sent out so-called "registration forms" as early as September 1939 to nearly all psychiatric institutions, hospitals, and nursing homes in which potential candidates were stationed. Helpful for the general registration as well as the basic success of the campaign was additionally the fact that in the first year after the seizure of power a nationalization of some psychiatric institutions took place; 3 years later this already included 24 institutions (Chroust et al. 1989, p. 18f.; Kepplinger 2008, p. 67; furthermore Debus et al. 1996, p. 44f.; Schmidt v. Blittersdorff et al. 1996, p. 70f.).

The reporting forms contained several queries about the home patients, which were constructed with a view to a possible selection. On the basis of this information, it should be possible to estimate the costs incurred or still to be incurred by the respective patient. Questions were asked, among other things, about the previous length of stay, the need for care or the (in-)ability to work (Aly 2013, pp. 43f., 60, 213f.; Klee 1986, p. 95f.). The true reason behind these recordings was not known to the persons in charge of the respective institutions who filled out the questionnaires, at least at the beginning of the action (Klee 1986, p. 92; Lifton 1988, p. 74; see for similar experiences in the Bavarian institution Kaufbeuren, Schmidt et al. 2012). Karl Rücker, who was once in charge of asylum matters in Kassel and who, among other things, had to take care of those forms together with other asylum directors, describes his experiences in the Hadamar trial:

---

[18] In fact, the abbreviation "T4" is not a National Socialist camouflage designation, but an acronym attributed from the trials as well as research of the post-war period for the centrally controlled first (gas murder) phase. In many cases, however, the entire murder operation is subsumed under "Aktion T4". In contemporary sources, on the other hand, this term is rarely, if ever, used (Aly 2013, p. 46; Hinz-Wessels et al. 2005, p. 79, FN 1).

[19] Of these six institutions, only four were active at any one time (Friedlander 1997, p. 155f.). The murder centres were Grafeneck (active January 1940–December 1940), Brandenburg (winter 1939/1940–September 1940), Bernburg (September 1940–August 1943), Hartheim (May 1940–December 1944), Sonnenstein (June 1940-Summer 1942 or 1943) and Hadamar (January 1941–August 1941 and August 1942–1945) (Hinz-Wessels et al. 2005, p. 91; Kepplinger 2008, p. 67).

In the beginning, we thought that these were the usual statistics that were asked for on a continuous basis, so to speak. [...] At that time the message came back from Berlin that the documents had to be filled out, that it was a matter of planned economic measures, that is, a better utilization of the available prison space; [...] We then heard nothing for months. And about the end of April 1941, the then Governor of the Land, Traupel, called the directors of the asylums and myself to him and said that he had now received news from Berlin according to which a generous planning for all asylums was in prospect, namely in such a way that certain groups of patients would be transferred to certain asylums. [...] In these institutions the sick would be examined again by a commission of doctors from Berlin, and would then be transferred to various institutions according to their abilities and their work assignments. He mentioned that it was not impossible that some of the sick, who were completely incurable, might, on the basis of the examination by the medical commission, be removed in a painless way, freed from their suffering, some of them. [...] When studying the questionnaires, our directors had established that it was essentially focussing on such sick persons for whom the prognosis for recovery was not very favourable, or for whom the capacity for work was not indicated as being so great. (statement by Rücker, witness, HHStA/a, p. 174ff.)

Insofar as the respective directors denied the question of the possibility of permanent and independent employment of the persons concerned, this was tantamount to (almost) irrevocably setting in motion the death sentence for the corresponding patient (Kneuker and Steglich 1985, p. 80ff.). The completed report forms were sent back to the T4 headquarters, where they were each passed on to three "medical experts". Based on their evaluations, they made a recommendation with regard to the question of life or death of the respective people without ever having seen them, with the potential exception of a few attached pictures. Finally, a single, hierarchically superior chief assessor was the final and thus commanding authority to decide on the measures to be taken. From this ongoing procedure, regular patient lists developed, which were to form the basis for the transport of the sick (Debus et al. 1996, p. 51; Hinz-Wessels et al. 2005, p. 87; Klee 1986, p. 97f.; Schmidt-von Blittersdorff et al. 1996, p. 102f.). In the catchment area of the Hadamar asylum, these reporting forms went out for the first time in June 1940, so that the T4 Central Office could prepare early and detailed plans for the murders, which did not begin until January 1941 (Schmidt-von Blittersdorff et al. 1996, p. 84).

After the data had been processed, the patients "to be euthanized" were first transported from their original institutions to so-called "intermediate institutions" (*Zwischenanstalten*). In addition to concealing the transport of patients, the system of intermediate institutions served, in particular, to plan and handle matters more effectively, both in an economic sense and for the purpose of further selection and culling of those eligible for action (Birkenfeld et al. 2017, p. 9; Lilienthal 2006a, p. 158f.; Roer 1992; instructive still Hinz-Wessels et al. 2005, p. 85ff.). Certainly, the system of intermediate institutions also created the additional option of being able to react appropriately to any resistance. Those involved with the admitted sick were thus granted an (informal or unofficial) "intervention period" (Aly 2013, p. 281), which, provided it was exercised with appropriate commitment, arguably created an opportunity to withdraw the respective patients from the impending transport to the gassing facility (ibid., pp. 69, 281). However, possible interventions were made more difficult by different (mostly administrative) measures, as is made clear, for example, by the withholding of outgoing letters from the patients (ibid., p. 89f.) or fundamental visiting bans (Sandner 2003, pp. 488, 507). In general, communication between the respective facility and the relatives was such that it either did not take place at all, or all information and notifications (e.g. about the patient's transfer and condition) were passed on with such delay and imprecision that it was hardly possible to follow the circumstances (Lilienthal 2006a, p. 159ff.; Sandner 2003, pp. 442ff., 489ff.; Schmidt-von Blittersdorff et al. 1996, pp. 95f., 114f.).

Thus, once they had entered Hadamar or another murder institution, only very few people still had any hope of survival. From the arrival of the patients to their murder and the subsequent post-processing of the deaths, the procedures followed a predetermined and systematic, above all bureaucratic, sequence. Soon the relatives received a standardized "comfort letter" announcing the death of the sick person along with the (fictitious) cause of death. The creation and recording of a supposedly natural cause of death should appear credible from a medical point of view and not contradict the previous medical record (Aly 2013, p. 33; Klee 1983, p. 140ff, 1986, p. 119; Lifton 1988, p. 85). From then on, this invented cause of death was officially listed on the death certificate (Kepplinger 2008, p. 91f.; Klee 1983, p. 151ff.). Instead of the real date of death, however, a date 1–3 weeks later was entered in order to be able to collect care costs for longer – probably the biggest source of profit for the Central Office in Berlin during this period (Aly 1985a, p. 27f.; Sandner 2003, p. 491).[20]

The Hadamar asylum was the last killing facility to be established after the gas murders at Grafeneck ceased in December 1940. A short time later, the new killing facility in the basement was constructed in Hadamar, which consisted, among other things, of a gas chamber, a dissection room and two incinerators. The gas killings at Hadamar began on 13 January 1941 and ended abruptly, on or around 21 August

---

[20] In the case of Jewish patients, the period was extended to (at least) 3–6 weeks, if not several months (Hinz-Wessels et al. 2005, p. 93f.; Lilienthal 2009, p. 6).

1941 (Debus et al. 1996, p. 53; Lilienthal 2006a; Schmidt-von Blittersdorff et al. 1996, pp. 82 ff; the subsequent period is addressed in Chap. 4, 5 and 6). In that year, the institution recorded the most victims of all euthanasia sites: 10,072 of the total of over 70,200 gassed patients lost their lives in Hadamar alone (followed by the Bernburg institution with 8601 victims, Klee 1986, p. 232; Schmidt-von Blittersdorff et al. 1996, p. 59; Schmuhl 2011c, p. 224).

Research Agenda: On Organized Brutalities

While the previous section merely referred to a forthcoming study within organizational sociology, the theoretical classification and analytical basis of this contribution should be specified here in view of the immense scope of the paradigm (see, for example, Apelt and Wilkesmann 2015; Tacke 2010). The research approach pursued is based on the fundamental assumption that the behaviour and actions of people within an organisational context change or can change in a direction desired by the organisation, or, even more precisely: can *be* changed. According to this assumption, organizations are able, by using certain means, to induce selected individuals to engage in – sometimes more, sometimes less detailed – defined activities that they would not, and in many cases could not, do away from such collective involvement (see, for example, Adams and Balfour 2009; Balcke 2001; Card 2005).

The point of the argument lies in the fact that such an analysis does not have to refer to extraordinary mechanisms tailored to an abnormal killing organization. On the contrary, reference is made to normal, downright typical processes as well as structures in and of organizations, which members can also – or especially – adopt when carrying out (genocidal) atrocities (for relevant elaborations of systems theory in this regard, see Kühl 2005, 2007b, 2014a). Of central importance in this context is the notion of organizations, which can be defined according to Luhmann's systems theory as a social system based on membership (especially Luhmann

1995; but instructive for the present work also Luhmann 2018a, c).[1] Within the framework of Luhmann's distinction between the three system types interaction, organization and society, the research interest is logically based on the level of the organizational system (Luhmann 2005; also Kühl 2014b).

To specify this in a paragraph in a more theoretically abstract sense, social systems are commonly spoken of as soon as the actions or communications of several people relate to each other in a meaningful way and the respective social order can be demarcated from an external, i.e. non-member, environment (Luhmann 1995, p. 23f., 2005, p. 10, 2018b, p. 135). A defining feature of social systems, then, includes a stable (internal) order or structure, which is characterized by a relative invariance to its environment on the one hand, and the concomitant relative independence of its own boundaries on the other (Luhmann 1983, p. 59, 1995, pp. 23f., 41, 2018c, p. 396). Simply put, a differentiation can be drawn according to the *interior* – meaning the system itself, respectively the internal order of the system – as well as the *exterior* (namely the environment) of the system (Luhmann 1995, p. 24, 2018b, p. 135).[2] In this context, an environment, irrespective of the respective system type, basically always offers more possibilities of action and experience than the corresponding system is able to process, or even perceive at all. A central func-

---

[1] I thus share the view not to indulge in the "deflationary tendencies" (Tacke 2015, p. 280) of the concept of organization (similarly Kühl 2015; Schimank 2015, p. 300f.). A counter-example from the recent past would be Ahrne and Brunsson's (2011; further Ahrne et al. 2016) notion of the "partial organization", in which, on the basis of five (seemingly arbitrarily selected) central features of the organization – membership, hierarchy, rules, monitoring and sanctions (Ahrne and Brunsson 2011, p. 85ff.) – a process of "(re-)organizing" is described in the case of all kinds of social structures and entities in order then interpret them as either complete or partial organizations (Tacke 2015, p. 286). However, the analytical value of this approach seems – at least from a systems theory perspective – to lie less in an organization theory analysis than in the explanation of certain transition processes from the system type of the group to the organization. When, for example, start-ups emerge from initial groups of friends and these companies become increasingly professionalized and standardized, (stricter) expectations regarding membership, hierarchy, rules, monitoring, and/or sanctions could be observed – according to a first assumption. Such an analysis, however, would be incumbent on a work based on sociological considerations about (peer-)groups (for a first introduction, see, for instance, Kühl 2019b; Neidhardt 1979, 1983).

[2] It should be noted here that the concept of environment does not only refer to external social units, but as a rule an internal environment must also be taken into consideration (Luhmann 2018c, p. 396). The latter is constituted by the simple fact that people are or can be part of the system only with selected, but not with all their actions and communications (Luhmann 2018c, pp. 396, 401; see also Barnard 1938, p. 65ff.): "Social systems do not consist of concrete persons with body and soul, but of concrete actions. [...] All persons, including the members, are therefore environment for the social system" (Luhmann 1995, p. 25).

tional feature of social systems, however, lies in the possibility of reducing precisely this complexity through processes of selection, so that only a few, but above all, *selected* possibilities of action and experience need to be considered (Luhmann 2005, p. 10, 2018c, p. 393ff.). The type of system in focus in this study, i.e. the organization, succeeds in this in particular through the generalization of (mostly relatively freely selected) formalized behavioral expectations, the acceptance of which is made a condition of membership for each member (Luhmann 1995, pp. 26, 41, 2018c, p. 393ff.).

This definition of the system type organisation, which is undoubtedly still somewhat unwieldy and seems almost typically clausulated for a system-theoretical approach, is to serve as the starting point for the following two sections. In the further course of the second chapter, these more abstract foundations will be elaborated in much greater detail and thus also "de-clausulized". This is relevant for the analysis of the eugenic campaign insofar as the systems-theoretical understanding of organizations functions in this work as an overarching framing, a kind of "master frame" under whose umbrella a multitude of (organization-)theoretical concepts and ideas are united in order to finally relate them to the empirical object.[3]

2.1 Memberships and Formal Expectations: Conformity and Obedience

A basic introductory insight lies in the fact that organizations use the concept of membership to differentiate between the members belonging to them on the one hand and the external non-members on the other (Luhmann 1995, p. 39ff., 2005, p. 13f.). In this context, memberships are not distributed randomly or unconsciously, but – in line with the "decision communication" specific to organizations – by conscious *decisions* that are made about who is, becomes, or may not (any longer) be part of the system (Luhmann 1995, p. 40f., 2005, p. 13f.; see also Kühl 2014b, p. 70, 2019a, p. 101f.).[4] The contingency of membership, i.e. the pos-

---

[3] I thank Thomas Hoebel for this reference.

[4] Of course, far from the organization there are other, so-called "membership-based systems", which can be (co-)determined by the characteristic of membership. In systems theory, one usually thinks of groups, families or (protest) movements (Kühl 2014b, a). In contrast to the latter, however, the membership issue in an organizational system is constituted not only as one, but as *the* central determinant par excellence (Kühl 2014b, p. 70). Furthermore, one can construct a substantive demarcation of these system types via the different communication possibilities or types – because in fact neither groups, nor families, nor movements use the decision communication mentioned (ibid., p. 69ff.).

sibility of entering and leaving the system based on voluntariness, is not so much an exception as a prerequisite and characteristic feature of organizations (Luhmann 1995, p. 41ff., 2005, p. 15, 2018a, p. 283, 2018c, pp. 395, 405). Unlike, for example, in families, where membership is a privilege conferred by birth or adoption and at the same time difficult to withdraw (Luhmann 1995, p. 41, 2018c, pp. 395), the organizational entry procedure is in most cases subject to self-selection by the member on the one hand – i.e. on a voluntary basis and as an "explicit act" (Tacke 2010, p. 348) – and to external selection by the organization on the other (Gruber 2017, p. 226; Kühl 2019a, p. 104; Luhmann 1995, p. 41).

On the basis of these provisions on membership, every organisation – and National Socialist violent organisations are no exception – has very specific *formal expectations* about what its members have to achieve. Through this (usually written) formality, each person's membership is bound to compliance with the respective requirements (Luhmann 1995, p. 39f., 2005, p. 13f.). In this regard, formal expectations are defined precisely by the fact that their non-observance or non-fulfilment cannot be reconciled with the continuity of membership (Luhmann 1995, pp. 38, 60). Behavioural expectations, which are summarized in the form of membership roles, are thereby primarily aligned with the respective concerns and desires of the social system (Luhmann 1995, pp. 35f., 46ff., 2018c, p. 395).[5] In addition to the blanket recognition of all organizational requirements and conditions, this also includes the acceptance of distributed tasks and competencies to all other members of the system (Luhmann 2018c, pp. 396, 399).

The consequence of this is that, through voluntary entry and the concomitant assumption of the membership role, a declared docility, i.e. a kind of obedience in principle, is performed on the part of the members, according to which they undertake to recognise and follow the set of rules referred to as formal expectations on a day-to-day basis and in its entirety – irrespective of whether these tasks present themselves as unfamiliar, uninteresting or unwanted (Gruber 2017, p. 226f.;

---

[5] A role is a bundle of (behavioural) expectations that is not fixed to specific people. Thus, even if the bearer of such a role varies, the behavioural expectations remain (largely) unchanged (Luhmann 1987, p. 84ff., 2018c, p. 394f.). In this sense, communication in an organization, at least insofar as it takes place on the basis of the formal role, is impersonal – although it can of course make a difference whether a role is filled by person A, B, or C (Gruber and Kühl 2015, p. 11; see also Luhmann 1995, p. 48). A forceful counter-example would be behavioural expectations that are addressed to individual persons, i.e. are shaped precisely by a person's personality, as is the case, for example, in families or groups of friends (Luhmann 1987, p. 85f., 1995, pp. 42f., 65f.).

Luhmann 1995, p. 36, 2018c, p. 399; Tacke 2010, p. 348f.).[6] Conversely, anyone who is unable to meet these behavioral requirements based on (at least apparent) consensus, or who openly rebels against them, is threatened with withdrawal from the member role, i.e. expulsion from the system (Luhmann 1995, pp. 35f., 2018c, pp. 394f.). Accordingly, members must continually ask themselves whether they behave appropriately – one could also say *correctly* – according to the prevailing formal rules (Luhmann 1995, pp. 36f., 42f., 2018a, p. 280). Formal expectations thus possess a veritable "monopoly on legitimacy" (Luhmann 2018a, p. 279), the recognition of which may not be refused and which are already valid by virtue of their entry without further ado (Luhmann 1995, pp. 35ff., 64, 2018a, pp. 279, 291).

Since *every* member must orientate himself or herself to these formalised expectations, it is ultimately secondary for the social system out of which motives the individual has actually joined and with which motivations the tasks are followed (Gruber and Kühl 2015, p. 11f.; Luhmann 1995, p. 41f., 2018c, p. 395). For ultimately, the formalization of membership expectations ensures that there is a generalized motivation of all members to comply with the system's internal requirements, however heterogeneous these may be in individual cases (Gruber and Kühl 2015, p. 11; Kühl 2014a, p. 241; Tacke 2010, p. 348f.). This structure is *generalized* in that every formal expectation exists independently of deviating individual events – i.e. it can also survive some disturbances or contradictions (Luhmann

---

[6] One can illustrate this with the example of an unsympathetic or uncharismatic superior: In spite of all professional or interpersonal incompetence, a member (in a hierarchically structured organization) has to accept the higher ranking as part of the formal order (Gruber 2017, pp. 226f., 232; Kühl 2011, pp. 34, 72; Luhmann 1995, p. 47). At the same time, said superior can be largely indifferent to the appreciation he or she receives because his or her orders are inherently legitimized by the formal hierarchical structure (including the accompanying formal status of the superior) (Gruber 2017, p. 227f.; Luhmann 1995, p. 96ff., 209, 2018a, p. 282ff.). The fact that there are, meanwhile, multiple possible informal ways of counteracting this network of relations in one way or another – one need only to think here of the supervision of the superior (Luhmann 1995, p. 273, 2018d) – is undoubtedly true, but irrelevant for the progress of this paper. In general, for analytical reasons, I address in this work almost exclusively formal structures and the associated behavioral expectations, which, it should be explicitly mentioned at this point, of course form only a part of the entire organizational action system (Luhmann 1995, p. 268ff.). Informal, i.e. norm-deviating, behaviour is nothing unusual in organisations – quite the contrary (Luhmann 1995, pp. 27f., 39, 48f., 283ff.; see also Sect. 3.4). The discovery of the "informal organization" is precisely the historical starting point of organizational sociology (Luhmann 1995, p. 29f.; Tacke and Drepper 2018, p. 16ff.).

1995, p. 55f.). In systems theory terms, this is referred to as the *generalization of behavioral expectations* (Luhmann 1995, p. 59f., 2018a, p. 277; see also Kühl 2014a, p. 240f.).[7]

The benefit for the organisation is obvious: in this way, conformity and obedience can be created to a high degree without having to constantly re-question or re-examine these properties in individual cases (Luhmann 1995, pp. 42, 61ff.). Ultimately, after all, an organization can declare all "what it considers good and important to be a condition of membership" (Kühl 2011, p. 32).[8] As long as the members want to keep their membership status, they have to actually follow the expectations set by the system (Tacke 2010, p. 348) – because even the breaking of a single rule may be considered a violation of all formal expectations (Kühl 2011, p. 33; Luhmann 1995, pp. 60, 63). Consequently, due to the generalization as well as formalization of membership motivations or expectations described here, a purpose or goal identification with the organization is not necessarily crucial for following instructions, but of course it is associated with considerable advantages, especially in violent organizations (Kühl 2014a, p. 239ff.). We will see later that the recruitment of personnel at the Hadamar murder centre was essentially based

[7] One is immediately inclined to run this idea through people who try to present as little personal involvement as possible in the context of their employment and thus maintain role distance as far as possible (Kühl 2014a, p. 225ff.; on the distinction between "personal" and "official roles", see, among others, Luhmann 1995, pp. 40, 63ff., 287). But of course the temporal, factual, and socially generalized formal order (detailed in Luhmann 1995, p. 54ff.) applies equally and in the same way to highly motivated members who fully identify with the purpose of the organization or the desirability of the acts performed within it. If, for example, an employee of Hadamar Institution had helped out in Pirna Institution on his or her own initiative because this would have seem useful to him or her, this behaviour would have led to great irritation not only at both institutions but also at the Berlin Central Office and, in all likelihood, to formally imposed sanctions for said member (for this, see also Kühl 2014a, p. 241f.).

[8] There are, of course, exceptions to this. An organization that acts completely detached from all rule deviations would inevitably fall into the bureaucratic or organizational nightmare of "work to rule" (Kieserling 2012, p. 131f.; Kühl 2007a, p. 270f., 2020a, p. 11; Osrecki 2015, pp. 17f., 20f.), a concept at least similar to the recently discovered trend of "Quiet Quitting". This is referred to, for example, by the notion of „Useful Illegality"coined by Niklas Luhmann (1995, p. 304ff.), according to which a behavior is informal or illegal, but the respective organization does not intervene because the end result of such a practice produces a significant advantage for it (detailed in Kühl 2020a). Taking into account the fact that the euthanasia was de facto illegal and a functionality for the National Socialist leadership can also be discerned, the killing program might thus be viewed from this perspective as well, if necessary. A further, conceptually similarly arranged exception can be found in the so-called "Prinz-von-Homburg-Effect" (Bosetzky 2019, p. 37ff.).

on factors that ensured a far-reaching congruence of purpose between personnel and organisation, or at least did not run counter to this (Sects. 3.3 and 6.1.3).

In principle, however, not all tasks or behaviors to which members commit themselves when joining an organization are prescribed or specified down to the smallest detail (Luhmann 1995, pp. 48, 93, 2018c, p. 397). This is related to the trivial fact that many tasks cannot be (adequately) represented for all kinds of reasons or should not be represented at all (Kühl 2011, p. 35; Luhmann 1995, pp. 85, 94). Instead, a rather rough or abstract "framework contract" is agreed upon between the organization and the respective member, which recurs to the aforementioned blanket recognition of all kinds of formally decided competences in the system (Gruber and Kühl 2015, p. 17; Luhmann 1995, p. 93f., 2018c, p. 397). In Hadamar, this can be seen in the fact that, with the exception of a smaller grouping, none of the hired members had initially been adequately told the full extent of the (killing) expectations placed upon them (Sandner 2003, pp. 419ff., 440f.; Wettlaufer 1996, p. 296). This exception is the so-called "Berlin staff", who were transferred to Hadamar after the Grafeneck asylum, where this collective had previously worked, was closed. Interestingly, however, it can be ascertained in the case of the Berlin staff that they were also not informed in an appropriate manner about the activities in the context of the interviews held before their first acquisition to Grafeneck (Wettlaufer 1996, pp. 295f., 319).

In this context, how can such a high level of compliance be explained, both theoretically and empirically, among (almost) all members?

2.2   On the Concept of the Zone of Indifference

Whether or not a particular task assigned to the member by the organization is taken on depends primarily on whether it is included by the membership and by the aforementioned framework contract that arises upon joining the organization. If such is the case, the instruction can be seen as a blanket matter of course despite its non-articulation (Gruber 2015, p. 37f.; Gruber and Kühl 2015, p. 17f.).

If certain expectations that have not been formulated are accepted by the member and not even questioned, they fall into the so-called "indifference zone" (Barnard 1938, p. 168ff.; Luhmann 1995, p. 96; also Gruber and Kühl 2015, p. 16ff.). In this sphere, a high degree of change, both positively and negatively, can be tolerated (Kühl 2005, p. 102f.; Luhmann 1995, p. 94f.). If, on the other hand, the opposite case exists with regard to questions concerning the willingness of members to accept and execute, the expectation of action is therefore *not* covered by the framework contract, the member will in all probability reject the task (see also

Brief et al. 2001, p. 479). Finally, the area between these two extremes exists in this context: The grey area, where as an organizational member one cannot be sure whether the instructions are covered by the organizational contract or not (Gruber and Kühl 2015, p. 18; Kühl 2005, p. 103).

In the remainder of this study, I will contradict hasty conclusions that place the National Socialist murders of the sick in this theoretical framework in the zone of indifference of the members of the organization from the very beginning – for example, due to alleged sadistic personality structures of the personnel. Instead, taking into account the empirical material, I would like to argue that the acts, especially in their early days – that is, before a certain routine could be established (see Sect. 3.1) – can be assigned to the grey area.

Ernst Klee (1986, p. 94) already explicitly pointed out that the perpetrators of euthanasia by no means corresponded to the ideas of the brutally acting excees, that they functioned as such but were ultimately not programmed as such (see also Hoffmann 2010). Numerous reports from the staff stationed in Hadamar confirm this assumption. Especially at the beginning, many of those involved harboured doubts about the permissibility of the killings, both in a legal and in a moral or ethical sense (Wettlaufer 1996, p. 307ff.). In this context, the actors repeatedly referred in statements and conversations to intense, above all psychologically stressful difficulties and concerns about the killings, as the following statements indicate:

I… looked through the peephole in the side wall… Through it I saw about 40 to 45 men who were crowded together in the next room and who were now slowly dying. […] The manner of death was so agonizing that one could not speak of a humane killing, especially since many of those killed may have had lucid moments. I watched the process for about 2–3 min and then moved away because I could no longer bear the sight and I felt sick. (statement by Lindner, office staff, quoted from Klee 1986, p. 125)

I saw through the window once, but not during the gassing, as long as a doctor was there, but only afterwards, when the doctor was gone. […] I felt the psychological effect on me well. I perished from this thing. Why? My wife can confirm that in 1940 I was always sitting at home and crying. When I looked at the children, I began to cry. (The defendant cries). Afterwards alone, when I continued to accompany my children downstairs and saw that they had gone the same way as the first ones, that really got me down. (statement by Härtle, nursing staff, HHStA/a, p. 71).

Attended the gassing? Unfortunately, yes. […] There were sick people in the room, naked people, some of them half slumped over, others with their mouths terribly wide open, their chests working. I saw that, I never saw anything more horrible. I went around, up the stairs again, there was a lavatory upstairs. Everything I had eaten I threw up. For days I was haunted by it, I must have talked about it at night, my wife held it against me. If you looked in there, I couldn't imagine that it was completely painless. (statement Lindner, office staff, HHStA/a, p. 125)

Finally, female nurses in particular expressed surprise and shock at the extent of the killings in Hadamar (Lilienthal 2006b, p. 285ff.; Wettlaufer 1996, pp. 307f., 319, 323f.), while Hubert Gomerski, the Hadamar corpse burner, referred to nausea and sleep disturbances resulting from his work (Klee 1986, p. 122, 126ff.; Lilienthal 2006b, p. 283f.).[9]

This brief excerpt from the empirical material, which can also be found in a very similar form for members of other murder institutions (see, for example, Klee 1986, p. 117; also Hoffmann 2010), already indicates that participation in the campaign was by no means unproblematic or self-evident. Participation in the mass murder activities was thus not per se in the zone of indifference, but was rather to be located in the grey area in which compliance with the instructions is on the one hand not clearly covered, but on the other hand can just as little be completely ruled out (Gruber 2015, p. 40). However, the fact that the acts could ultimately leave the area of indeterminacy and even be established as a blanket expectation is due to the dynamic boundaries of the zone of indifference.[10]

Classically, the influencing and expansion of the zone of indifference is described as a possibility available only to the authority side. Accordingly, the member-side zone of indifference is static (Barnard 1938, p. 167ff.). I argue instead for the contrary assumption of a fundamentally dynamic conception of the zone of indifference, in which the transitions between the individual zones are fluid. In this way, it becomes comprehensible how participation in mass murder could be institutionalized as a condition of membership that was increasingly taken for granted, in defiance of all individual obstacles there may have been. In this context, it was both the mechanisms and structures introduced and implemented by the organization – i.e. the expansion of the zone of indifference by the authority side – and any strategies employed by the members – the member-side shifting of the zone of indifference – that led to a unified process of the killings (Sects. 3.1–3.3). As a result, there has been a *normalization of illegal practices* (Ashforth and Anand 2003), which, taking into account the dynamic boundaries of the zone of indifference, has led to the acts becoming established as indifferent and legitimate expectations among institutional staff.

---

[9] While it has already been explicitly mentioned that the nursing staff was not trained to become mass murderers, the same naturally applies to the burners. In the case of this group in particular, there is evidence to suggest that their complicity could hardly have belonged to a zone of indifference that existed from the outset, since before their tasks as burners they usually pursued skilled trades and/or administrative and office jobs (Klee 1986, pp. 122, 124; Lilienthal 2006b, p. 283).

[10] The understanding of the zone of indifference used below no longer follows the classical static notion of the concept developed by Barnard (1938, p. 168ff.), but is reinterpreted in a systems-theoretical sense in line with the theoretical framing of this paper (on this, Gruber and Kühl 2015, p. 17ff.; Kühl 2007b, p. 18f.).

On the Normalization of Illegal Practices

3

The notion of the normalization of illegal practices in organizations after Ashforth and Anand (2003) helps to explain how seemingly morally upright people can regularly engage in corrupt or illegal acts without coming into major conflict with themselves (ibid., p. 1).[1] In relation to the first phase of murder, an explanation is sought in this way as to how it was possible not only to legitimize and stabilize the (co-)participation of the foot soldiers of euthanasia, but how the acts ultimately became routine, and in this framework were sometimes even considered desirable. Following the model's baseline, the subsequent explanations are divided into the

---

[1] In many cases, the studies centrally referenced for the further analysis of the first (Chap. 3) and second (Chap. 6) murder phases do not address genocides, let alone Nazi euthanasia. As a rule, the research interest of most used literature concerns organizational white-collar crime (see especially the studies on the concept of normalization, Ashforth and Anand 2003; Brief et al. 2001; Gioia 1992; further Anand et al. 2004; Ashforth and Kreiner 1999; Kaptein and van Helvoort 2018; with closer reference to the object of study, Adams and Balfour 2009; Bandura 1990). My approach of using some of the central premises of these contributions is not to trivialize the euthanasia action, but instead to address the complex nature of the object of study with the method of analogical comparison often used in sociology. In this sense, I attempt to "explain a social event that is puzzling in at least one respect with the help of sociological insights about another specific social event" (Hoebel 2018, p. 178). Such an analogical approach is helpful insofar as the ideas that are transferred (and, if necessary, slightly modified in the process) are, as a rule, largely elaborated, consequently rather convincing from the outset (Abbott 2004, p. 114ff.; Hoebel 2018, p. 178f.).

institutionalization (Sect. 3.1), the rationalization (3.2), and the socialization of (new) members into the unlawful acts (Sect. 3.3).[2]

The elaborated argumentative three-step approach is primarily to be understood as an analytical separation; it can already be seen from the (simplified) visual representation of the model (see Ashforth and Anand 2003, p. 3) that the three pillars of normalization are not to be understood as distinctive, but as influencing as well as mutually reinforcing social processes (see also Brief et al. 2001, p. 473). At the same time, all three theoretical pillars – i.e. institutionalization, rationalization as well as socialization – are necessary for the normalization of illegal practices (Ashforth and Anand 2003, pp. 3, 34). In this respect, the boundaries between the pillars in social reality may be fluid and not as clear-cut as the model suggests at first glance. The analysis will reveal numerous (more or less) direct interactions and overlaps of that kind at various points. Furthermore, in the concluding chapter of this section, I will go into more detail on some overlaps and the implications to be drawn from them, in order to finally present empirically supported objections (Sect. 3.4).

At the beginning of this study (Sect. 1.1), I pointed out that illegal practices and, in the broadest sense, thereby also organized brutalities are usually based on the cooperation of many or all members of the institutions. The same applies to the euthanasia institutions, including Hadamar. Of course, it cannot and should not be excluded that there were isolated outliers and, at the latest with the beginning of the killings, also differentiated positions on the activities within the institution(s), but these considerations play at most a secondary role in the present framework and its line of argumentation. This conclusion is not only convincing in a more theoretical-abstract sense due to the already presented generalization of membership motivations as well as the formalization of behavioral expectations (Chap. 2), but is also reflected in the empirically reconstructed participation in mass murder, in which the forms of participation varied between half-hearted and proactive murder. Despite the apparent inconsistencies between nursing professional ethics and the murders of the sick, there were never any forms of open resistance (see, for example, Roer and Henkel 1996b, p. 31f.).

---

[2] This does not mean, however, that the structure presented by Ashforth and Anand (2003) is adopted without exception beyond this initial decomposition. If appropriate, there are abridgements and mergers of some aspects. Helpful are other writings that follow a similar line of argument (Ashforth and Kreiner 1999; Anand et al. 2004). In particular, the analytical strand of neutralization or rationalization strategies can be complemented by analogous accounts (especially Kaptein and van Helvoort 2018; Sykes and Matza 1957).

3.1   The Institutionalization of the Killings

Institutionalized behaviors and actions in organizations are defined as very stable, repetitive and long-lasting activities that are performed by a larger group of members. It is characteristic of such processes that they are practiced routinely and thus in a certain sense without deliberation, i.e. the actors carrying them out do not have to or should not think about their (moral) correctness or actual usefulness. Strictly speaking, the implementation of the procedures does not even depend on the moral or ethical consent of the agents (Ashforth and Anand 2003, p. 4; Brief et al. 2001, p. 481). In this context, the processual procedure of institutionalization begins with an initial stage, which is intended to create the basis for the (here: murderous) routines that will be discussed later (Ashforth and Anand 2003, p. 4ff.; also Adams and Balfour 2009, p. 24). In this initial stage, the origins of illegality are still at stake. During this time, framework conditions are created that not only favour or set in motion the genesis of rule-deviating practices, but also ascribe a fundamentally legitimate, or at least not immoral, character to them (Ashforth and Anand 2003, p. 5ff.; further Adams and Balfour 2009, p. 27).[3]

In the case of eugenic campaign, however, it is difficult to determine a starting point based on general consensus. With every determination, the objection could inevitably be raised that one could or even should have gone back further for an analysis. Martin Weißmann (2015, p. 81ff.), in his study of dehumanization in genocides, draws attention to the fact that such processes usually have a long history and that they can undoubtedly facilitate mass killings, even if not necessary. But how exactly is one to determine at what point a eugenic movement is perceived as relevant enough to mark it as the beginning of an investigation?

From a sociological perspective, it can be emphasized that the selection and justification of a relevant starting point, as is common in argumentation emphasizing temporal structure, must be done analytically (Ashforth and Anand 2003, p. 41; Falleti and Mahoney 2015, p. 214ff.; Pierson 2003, p. 149). In the present context, then, the initial aim is to identify decisions, actions or more general frameworks that contributed significantly to an acceptable ethical climate at the societal and/or organizational level and thereby possessed initiatory character for the genesis as well as subsequent legitimation of the illegal practices (Ashforth and Anand 2003, p. 5; further Luft 2020, p. 320f.).

---

[3] Welzer (2005) describes a fundamentally similar idea with regard to some episodes of the Holocaust when he speaks of a shift in the frame of reference and the particularistic, National Socialist (killing) morality that forms within it (for this discussion, see also Christ 2014, p. 334, FN 2).

The events of 1933 and 1934 form an emphatically meaningful starting point for euthanasia because at this time the initiation of the later murders can be observed on two different levels at once. On the one hand, the discussion about the right to life of the allegedly incurably ill found increasing relevance as well as participation at the societal level (Faulstich 1998, p. 103; Kaiser et al. 1992, p. 210ff.; also Kühl 1994, pp. xiii ff., 27ff., 35ff.). An originally small racial hygiene movement expanded more and more, not least in view of an accompanying "scientification" (Schmuhl 2011a, pp. 28f., 2011c, p. 217). On the other hand, this period also saw the first – but by no means the last (see, for example, Friedlander 1997, pp. 61f., 65ff.; Sandner 2003, p. 240) – official and legally secured deformation and stigmatization of the sick (Chroust et al. 1989, p. 14ff.; Debus et al. 1996, p. 39f.; Kaiser et al. 1992, p. 126ff.; Schmuhl 2011b), which received widespread social approval (Kühl 1994, pp. 38ff., 48ff.; Bryant 2005, p. 24ff.; Kaiser et al. 1992, p. 160ff.): "Thus the state intervenes in the life of the individual, destroys his procreative capacity, if his hereditary masses are detrimental to the overall national growth" (Höhn 1934, p. 24).[4] With these provisions, a first verbal genocide begins towards the people who will be the focus of the later operation: the following acts of violence were ultimately a consequence of National Socialist political leader-

---

[4] The personal case of Reinhard Höhn, a lawyer and SS-Oberführer relevant to political science at the time, is of interest far from the context presented here because Höhn was able to pursue a significant career in the twilight of his National Socialist past. Höhn was the founder of the so-called "Harzburg Model," a management program that was probably the first in the Federal Republic of Germany to deal with a systematization of leadership and leadership theory. It was considered one of the most widespread management concepts until the mid-1970s (most prominently, see Höhn 1969). As time went on, historians in particular pointed to (supposed) similarities between Höhn's Harzburg Model on the one hand and National Socialist operational structures on the other: Höhn had, according to a phrase often used in this debate, continued old operational structures in a "denazified" version, and everyone had fallen for it (for example, Wildt 2011). In my view, however, it is not unlikely that a view informed by organizational sociology would come to a different conclusion. In this respect, the question of substantive continuities and ruptures does not seem to have been conclusively clarified at this point in time due to the lack of sociological (counter-)perspectives. An introduction to the debate can be found in Firkus (2021).

ship, but it cannot be denied that the political leadership was elevated to a form of violence itself (Christ 2014, pp. 332, 337, 348).[5]

In addition, at about the same time or concomitantly, in view of an enormous austerity policy in the field of psychiatry, the already scarce financial resources available were even further decreasing for the state sanatoria, especially in Hessen-Nassau and Hadamar (Faulstich 1998, pp. 101ff., 212f., 237f., 540ff.; Sandner 2003, p. 270ff., 2006, p. 141f.; Roer and Henkel 1996b). The simultaneous nationalization of the asylums (Sect. 1.3) led to a significant increase in the number of patients, which inevitably resulted in overcrowded rooms with extremely poor conditions for the sick and a simultaneous shortage of personnel. The latter problem was of course intensified by the subsequent military conscription of many men (Faulstich 1998, p. 245f.; Sandner 2006, p. 142). At any rate, the supply and general survival of many patients could no longer be guaranteed even at this early stage (Chroust et al. 1989, p. 25; Daum 1996, pp. 186ff., 199ff.; Roer and Henkel 1996b, p. 23f.; Schmidt-von Blittersdorff et al. 1996, p. 74ff.). In fact, over time and especially in the context of the second murder phase, starvation became an increasingly important factor in psychiatric institutions (for a detailed discussion, see Faulstich 1998; see also Sect. 6.1.4). The new pro-ideological content of the training did the rest in illustrating the worthlessness of the sick, which was oriented towards a combination of racial ideology and economic aspects, in order to create or legitimize the framework conditions for the whole initiative (Wettlaufer 1996, p. 292ff.; see also Sect. 3.2.6).[6]

Once the point of such a legitimizing structure is reached, the implementation of the illegal practices can easily begin – all that is needed is an opportunity that seems appropriate or suitable to set the procedure in motion (Ashforth and Anand

---

[5] Bryant (2005, p. 14ff.) chooses the experience and traumatic consequences of the First World War in the early 1920s as his starting point for contextual incorporation, pointing out that the combination of eugenic and racial hygienic ideas became a "potent cocktail for many Germans in the Weimar years" (ibid., p. 14) at this time. This was partly due to the fact that the defeat in the First World War had already been attributed to the allegedly already advanced decay of the German national body (Kneuker and Steglich 1985, p. 19f.; Schmuhl 2011a, p. 27f.). Bryant (2005, p. 15) outlines in his study that it was precisely in the following years that the actually relevant public statements, demands as well as legitimations regarding the eugenic movement occurred, whereby the voices advocating the eugenic solutions became particularly loud from the mid-1930s onwards – ultimately, therefore, a view that is shared in the present remarks.

[6] Such racial ideological or hygienic principles were also demonstrated to medical students, among others (Kaiser et al. 1992, p. 235; Schmuhl 2011a, p. 27f.; for a literature review on the "brown universities" and medical faculties, see Eckart 2011).

2003, p. 6). For this, if one recalls the initial dating of euthanasia, which is known to have occurred around or with the onset of war, one can clearly see the calculus behind the decision to implement the planned measures in the context of war (Bryant 2005, p. 27; Debus et al. 1996, p. 50; Klee 1983, p. 87). Appropriately, around 1935, Hitler is reported to have said in a conversation with the Reichsärzteführer at that time "that such a problem is initially smoother and easier to implement in wartime" (quoted in Chroust et al. 1989, p. 33; see also Mitscherlich and Mielke 1995, p. 237).

Once such an initial phase – including the associated introductory decision(s) – has been completed, there is, from a theoretical point of view, a second fundamental key factor that is of necessary relevance to the process of institutionalizing illegal practices: the aspect of leadership (Ashforth and Anand 2003, p. 6ff.). In this sense, superiors or those of higher rank do not necessarily have to behave in an exemplary manner in the sense of the illegal practices, but simply facilitate the success of the acts or even reward them. In the context of the euthanasia campaign, this was achieved, for example, through above-average monthly remuneration (Friedlander 1997, p. 375; Klee 1986, p. 124f.; Kneuker and Steglich 1985, pp. 27, 41f.), plus room and board for the staff (statement by Lindner, office staff, HHStA/a, p. 121; see also Sect. 3.2.3), as well as through numerous additional gratuities taken over by the T4 organisation. These included generally known and recognised allowances, such as Christmas and death bonuses or insurance payments (Sandner 2003, pp. 426, 432ff.), the opportunity to spend the provided holiday together in the T4 recreation home (Kepplinger 2008, p. 97; Sandner 2003, p. 464), but also supposedly smaller, informal gestures, such as the so-called silence or loyalty bonus payments or large quantities of alcohol (Kepplinger 2008, p. 97; Klee 1986, pp. 125, 130, 134; also Sect. 3.3).[7] Organisations that reward their members monetarily can generally expect a greater zone of indifference on their part than those organisations with other membership motivations (Kühl 2007b, p. 18, 2014a, p. 240; also Barnard 1938, p. 168f.; Brief et al. 2001, p. 479; for a list of common means of motivation, see Kühl 2011, p. 37ff.).

Beyond this, however, the decisive factor is that those higher up in the hierarchy are in a position to authorize the practices, so that the legitimate expectation can be

---

[7] Ashforth and Anand (2003, p. 7) point out that informal gratifications are neither unusual nor do they have a lesser effect than formal benefits. On the contrary, it can be argued that the labour of organisational members can be mobilised for particularly unattractive and/or officially prohibited behaviour precisely *through* informal commendations (Kühl 2020a, p. 76f.). This may also be the reason why the so-called loyalty or silence bonuses were issued in particular to the burners, who arguably had to perform the most demanding task, physically as well as psychologically, during the first murder phase (see Sect. 3.3).

placed on subordinates not only not to question these calls to action, but actually to carry them out (Ashforth and Anand 2003, p. 7; Brief et al. 2001, pp. 476f., 480; also Ermann and Lundman 1978, p. 57). At the time of the eugenic campaign, this point is highly significant because an enormously strong hierarchical relationship characterized the relations between doctors and nurses (Benedict 2003, p. 76; Hoffmann 2010, p. 255; Lilienthal 2006b, p. 286; Wettlaufer 1996, p. 306f.). Such unambiguous hierarchical structures are helpful with regard to the obedience of the members as well as the legitimation of the demands and actions – even or especially with regard to such instructions that the actors themselves, on a personal level far from their organizational involvement, would not tolerate (Ashforth and Anand 2003, p. 7; Brief et al. 2001, p. 478f.; Zimbardo 2009).[8] These assumptions are confirmed by, among others, nurse Paul Reuter several decades after the operation: Reuter pointed out that he had come to the conclusion at that time, after repeated statements by hierarchically higher-ups, that he

> was serving a merciful cause in this matter. I also had the impression at the beginning of my work. […] In my opinion, the gassing process lasted only three to four minutes and, when questioned, I was told by various people that a quicker elimination would not be possible. […] If I am now reproached for having actively participated in the elimination of the sick, I must confirm this. I realize today that at that time, blindly following obedience, I participated in the killing of the sick. (Kneuker and Steglich 1985, p. 28f.)

What is remarkable here, while at the same time complying with the argument, is that the former nurse acknowledges the illegal practices as such as soon as the authorization by those hierarchically higher up fails to materialize (Adams and Balfour 2009, p. 149; Ashforth and Kreiner 2002, p. 25f.; also Welzer 2005, p. 12f.). In a similar vein, nurse Zachow expressed that she had always held the motto that "if the doctor does it, it will not be cruel to the sick person" (quoted in Wettlaufer 1996, p. 307). In fact, a pronounced attitude of obedience can be observed among all euthanasia workers, but especially among the nursing staff (Wettlaufer 1996, p. 306ff.; for more details, see Sect. 3.2.3).

One might object at this point that in parts of the second chapter it was pointed out several times that the conformity of behaviour is ensured primarily via the membership conditions and the subsequent expanding zone of indifference,

---

[8] Ashforth and Anand trace this insight back to the Milgram experiment. In view of the already successful reinterpretation of this experiment in organizational sociology (see Kühl 2005, 2007b, c) as well as other experiments on obedience, the integration of the insights gained from it seems to be a logical connection.

whereas the focus has so far been on the hierarchy. However, this is not to be seen as a contradiction, but rather, within the framework of Luhmann's sociology of organization, as a thoroughly interrelated and interdependent function or consequence of formal organizations. It is precisely the acceptance of hierarchy that is regarded as a central condition of membership: Whoever is a member of an organization has to obey the orders of his superior, even if these are perceived as not too meaningful, as uninteresting, or as cruel (Balcke 2001, p. 81ff.; Kühl 2011, pp. 71, 84ff.). Accordingly, the legitimation of hierarchy helps to ensure that even unusual, sometimes inhumane demands can be recognized (Adams and Balfour 2009, p. xxxv; Kühl 2007b, p. 13) – which may even include, as the present case shows, the day-to-day burning of countless corpses despite prior manual training (Klee 1986, p. 124ff.; Lilienthal 2006b, p. 283f.). In the killing centres, it was thus the (rule-) conformists who were in the right in the event of conflict, while deviant as well as disobedient behaviour led or could lead to sanctions (Lilienthal 2006b, p. 284; see also Chap. 2) – the only difference being that in this case precisely the non-conformist behaviour would have been the proper alternative from a legal point of view (Campbell and Göritz 2014, p. 291f.).[9]

From this combination of the overall social and organizational conditions that arose in the initial period on the one hand, and the authority structures in the institution on the other, an increasing embedding of the illegal practices in the organizational processes and structures finally emerged: they became a habit not only in view of their legitimacy, but also because of their long-term and regular nature (Ashforth and Anand 2003, p. 8ff.; also Pinto et al. 2008, p. 692f.). Repetitive sequences of actions can be observed in abundance in the case study, especially in the repetitive sequence of killings in almost everyday practice (see, for example, Chroust et al. 1989, p. 46; Klee 1986, pp. 119, 124ff., 151 ff.; Lilienthal 2006a, p. 159ff.; Schmidt-von Blittersdorff et al. 1996, p. 89ff.): The bus transports of the patients drove into the wooden garage of the asylum as part of their arrival. The sick were taken through an airlock into a waiting room. From here they were taken

---

[9] As a result, the former Hadamar state sanatorium and the other euthanasia institutions represent, at least retrospectively, a peculiar hybrid form of "organized" and "organizational crime" (see Kühl 2020a, p. 48ff.; also Paul and Schwalb 2012). This hybrid form comes about because in the case of organized crime – for example, mafia-like associations –, violations of the law are expected to run counter to state claims, while in the context of organizational crime the state claim is formally accepted, but at the same time there are informal expectations to act close to or even beyond the boundaries of legality (Kühl 2020a, p. 49). In the context of eugenic action, violations of the law were expected on a formal level, which at the same time did not run counter to the state's claims, making it incompatible with both typifications (see also Ebbinghaus 2008, p. 215).

one by one to the undressing room before the nursing staff escorted them individually to the doctors' room. The examination by the doctors consisted of a final ap-
praisal of the person in order to be able to establish an official cause of death which
was to be carried along from then on and which did not have to be in contradiction
with the patient's previous medical record (Sect. 1.3). In extremely rare cases – i.e.
when it was determined that the patient was fit for work – the patients were, if
necessary, returned to the hospital.[10] In accordance with a more far-reaching
interest (with regard to research or the plundering of corpses), some sick people
were visually marked by coloured pencil marks on their backs (Lilienthal 2006b,
p. 278f.). After this final examination, patients were led to the photo room before
being gathered in a waiting room on the opposite side. When the entire group was
present, the individuals were led to the basement room where the gassing facility
was located. The doors were locked before the doctor controlled the gas supply
from an adjoining room. The chief physician of the first phase, Dr. Bodo Gorgaß,
described this pre-programmed killing process in his interrogation as follows:

> The sick were reexamined briefly after their arrival, photographed and then led to the
> shower room. It always took hours, as I saw in Hadamar and as it was carried out
> there. One by one they were led in. The patient's medical history and photocopy of the
> registration form were lying there. On the basis of these sheets the patient was ex-
> plored one last time. In the case of schizophrenic end states, in the case of feeble-
> mindedness, in most cases it does not require a further examination to determine the
> severity of the illness. [...] They came in undressed and were usually weighed before-
> hand. The examination lasted a few minutes on average. In case of profound imbecil-
> ity, any examination could be waived, as they hardly uttered any actual words. [...]
> When the examination was over? Then they were led into the shower room. [...] The
> process lasted a few minutes. There was also a window. I once looked through that
> window. How death occurred and so on? That was CO gas. It has a suffocating effect,
> not by external respiratory distress, but by the fact that a conversion takes place in the
> blood and leads to death by suffocation. The death is a peaceful one. It is a simple
> sleeping, in the truest sense of the word. People tire and lose all connection with the
> outside world and then fall asleep. (statement by Gorgaß, chief physician, HHStA/a,
> p. 13ff.)

After death, the room was vented of gas. The subsequent task of the burners was to
take the corpses out of the room and either burn them directly in the inmate crema-
toria, or alternatively to loot them beforehand according to the markings, or to bring

---

[10] Sandner (2003, p. 467) estimates the number of sick persons deferred in Hadamar in 1941
at less than 1 percent (see also Lilienthal 2006a, p. 161f.; Schmidt-von Blittersdorff et al.
1996, p. 92f.).

the medically exceptional cases to the dissection room for "scientific examination" (Burlon 2009, p. 25; Hinz-Wessels et al. 2005, p. 101ff.; Kepplinger 2008, p. 83f.).

During the entirety of the gas murder phase in Hadamar, which lasted about 8 months, almost nothing changed in this process. On the contrary, it can be stated that the transports arriving from the intermediate institutions arrived with such regularity that the murder machinery was "optimally utilized". Sometimes daily transports could be observed (Chroust et al. 1989, p. 53). In view of the marginal, if any, changes or adjustments to the procedure, which in view of their regularity became a daily repetitive procedure, the staff became accustomed to it (Schmidt-von Blittersdorff et al. 1996, p. 84ff.). From a certain point onwards, the killings were automated (Kneuker and Steglich 1985, p. 41ff.).

In view of the documentation and processing of basically all cases, the bureaucratically structured procedures can furthermore be observed in other parts of the institution (Chroust et al. 1989, pp. 44f., 47, 84ff.; Klee 1986, p. 137ff.). There were various internal statistics with correspondingly proper index cards, distinguishable by colour, for all T4 institutions (Sandner 1999, pp. 391, 393; Schmidt-von Blittersdorff et al. 1996, p. 97). The handling of patients who were already dead also followed a determined and bureaucratically time-consuming administrative act carried out for the purpose of concealment: Thus, an almost identical letter of consolation including a falsified cause of death – "That was a scheme, always in the same form, without variations" (statement Schmidt, office staff, HHStA/a, p. 119) – was sent out. This was followed by a subsequent shipment of urns, spiked with random ashes of the sick mixed from the human remains (Klee 1983, p. 150f., 1986, p. 119; Lilienthal 2006a, p. 162ff.; Sandner 2003, p. 625): "Several corpses went into one oven, simultaneously. [...] It is true that the people did not get the ashes of their deceased at all" (statement Gorgaß, chief physician, HHStA/a, p. 15). At the same time, standardized records of the valuables and clothing from the dead were kept as accurate and detailed as possible (Schmidt-von Blittersdorff et al. 1996, p. 95ff.). The defendant Bacher describes the bureaucratic handling of the gold teeth taken from the sick before they were burned:

> Gold teeth? They were given to us in the office if someone was there who had gold teeth. [...] One of the disinfectors brought them to me in a bowl. He had a book and I had a book, so we acknowledged each other and then we left them. We had a small box in which they lay until more came together, which we then sent to Berlin by courier. There was a regular courier service between Hadamar and Berlin and between the institutions in general. (statement by Bacher, office staff, HHStA/a, p. 148)

It can be concluded that, over time, the killing-related processes became not only habitual, but ultimately routine. This further development is to be classified as relevant as it inhibited the illegal and immoral character of the acts for the perpetrators in various ways (Ashforth and Anand 2003, p. 11ff.).

One manifestation of this can be found, for example, in the extensive reduction or negation of reflective thoughts in relation to the deeds (Ashforth and Anand 2003, p. 11; Campbell and Göritz 2014, p. 295). This way, such practices become *"recognition* rather than construction" (Ashforth and Fried 1988, p. 308, ed.). Accordingly, once Pauline Kneissler had familiarized herself with the killing work and overcome her initial horror, a real habituation effect can be observed (so Wettlaufer 1996, p. 319f.). Similarly, the nurse Paul Reuter mentioned earlier, stated that he had simply stopped worrying about the question why people who obviously did not meet the actual criteria for being murdered were not spared, for instance when they were still able to work (Kneuker and Steglich 1985, p. 28). Sister Zachow also gave an analogous explanation (Wettlaufer 1996, p. 308).

A second form of the abolition of the illegal character that follows from the routine arises as a result of the division of labor, which is exercised for the purpose of improving efficiency – or, in Hadamar, in the sense of a higher (killing) effectiveness. In such contexts, the participants usually refer to an account of the events according to which, in view of their small and insignificant contribution to the overall work, neither guilt nor responsibility could be attributed to them, and thus they sometimes even refer per se to their own impunity. Where appropriate, this logic is additionally applied to their own department or form of work (Ashforth and Anand 2003, p. 12; Brief et al. 2001, p. 480; Kaptein and van Helvoort 2018, p. 15f.). It is out of question that the Hadamar mass murder required a routine procedure based on the division of labor; in addition to the killing process already described, we only need to refer to the five different departments (transport, admissions, homicide, administration, as well as economic department) of the institution as examples (Lilienthal 2006b, p. 270). In particular, large sections of the office staff drew attention to their limited role in the overall procedure, because they had in fact little or no physical contact with the sick[11]:

I worked in the personnel department [...]. Did I see anything of the action? No, nothing. I didn't look at any rooms, didn't see any patients arriving. (statement by J. Thomas, office staff, HHStA/a, p. 128)

---

[11] Even if the reference to the limited role was useful as a responsibility-relieving mechanism for the office staff in particular, this does not rule out the possibility that the nursing staff could not be guided by a similar strategy. In the course of my elaboration on the rationalization strategies in the next chapter, I will discuss in detail the technique of "denial of harm" (Sect. 3.2.5), which was used by the nursing staff despite direct and physical contact with the sick in the gas murder phase.

My conscience did not need to come forward; I had done no criminal acts. I did not think what was done to the insane was right. [...] Reproached myself? No. [...] Did I think what I myself did was right? I did not do any criminal acts. (statement Lichtefellt, office staff, HHStA/a, p. 144)

I never experienced the gassing process. I never saw sick people when they came. [...] I never looked at the gassing room. I didn't want to see it at all, I always resisted it very much. I also never saw the unloading of the sick. (statement by Gerst, office staff, HHStA/a, p. 150)

Philipp Blum, who was first responsible for the telephone service and later the institution's cemetery caretaker, made similar comments long after the activities in Hadamar (technical staff, Kneuker and Steglich 1985, p. 45f.). Meanwhile, nurse Irmgard Huber, who had worked in the laundry room during the gas murder phase, not only drew attention to her lack of guilt and lack of participation in general (similarly nurse Schrankel with reference to her kitchen activities, HHStA/b, p. 21f.; additional similarities also in the case of Lückoff, nursing staff, HHStA/b, p. 22). Huber further emphasized that, given her professional position in the institution, she had noticed what was really going on only as time went on (statement Huber, nursing staff, HHStA/a, p. 48; Wettlaufer 1996, p. 322f.).[12] Indeed, on the basis of their limited role in the overall procedure, many of those involved point to a supposed lack of awareness to the true extent of the eugenic action or, alternatively, that this awareness only occurred at a time when it was already too late (thus the concluding assessment for the office staff in HHStA/b, pp. 23, 31 ff.; confirming also Weimer's statement, nursing staff, HHStA/a, p. 104; Gerst's statement, office staff, HHStA/a, p. 152; M. Schmidt's statement, office staff, HHStA/a, p. 119; as well as Blum's statement, technical staff, Kneuker and Steglich, 1985, p. 42; theoretical implications on this in Ashforth and Anand 2003, p. 12; Brief et al. 2001, p. 481f.; Kaptein and van Helvoort 2018, p. 17f.).

---

[12] The statements of Irmgard Huber in particular point to the problem of retrospective statements mentioned in Sect. 1.2. After all, it seems extremely questionable – to put it charitably – that Sister Huber would have needed a longer period of time to understand the full extent of the activities in the institution. Not only does it appear from the sources that she had her residence at the asylum in addition to her employment, but we know, moreover, of a longstanding emotional relationship with the then administrative inspector Alfons Klein (Wettlaufer 1996, p. 323f.): "I took care of this man, gave him money and supported him in every way. [...] I had pity for him and from pity to love it is not a long way. The love was returned by him" (statement Huber, nursing staff, HHStA/a, p. 245f.). After the end of the gassing phase, Irmgard Huber remained at Hadamar until the US troops marched in (March 1945), even rising to the position of head nurse during the second murder phase (Wettlaufer 1996, p. 324; Chap. 6).

If a certain interdependence in the work processes and thus among the prison staff had already arisen as a result of the separation of work, the members' need for social interaction with like-minded people increased even more as a result of the illegal practices. In accordance with the following increased exchange with each other, the illegal character of the acts is again reduced or minimized: "Aversive stimuli – such as perceptions of corrupt activity – foster a desire for social interaction for purposes of sense making, social support and anxiety relief" (Ashforth and Anand 2003, p. 14). In this context, intra-group solidarity is comparatively high, especially in organizations that, just like the Hadamar asylum, engage in "dirty work"[13] – "that is, widely shared and deeply held systems of values, beliefs and norms" (Ashforth and Kreiner 1999, p. 414) were developed (see also Ashforth and Anand 2003, p. 9f.; Bandura 1990, p. 36f.; Campbell and Göritz 2014, p. 292). Such heightened internal connectedness is simultaneously accompanied by a distinct separation from all other social circles far from the organization. This specifically undertaken segregation and exclusion is thereby all the greater, the more the respective individuals socialize with their colleagues (Ashforth and Kreiner 1999, p. 420).

Accordingly, the categorization of the procedures that took place in the murder institutions as "dirty work" appears to be extremely apt, not only in view of the murderous practices, but because this description can also be reproduced in terms of the generally low standing and the accompanying social stigmatization of the nurses working in the field of psychiatry. Sometimes, in view of these circumstances, an (un-)conscious distancing as well as a lack of solidarity between the nurses and the patients on the one hand, and a much greater sense of belonging among themselves on the other, can be observed (Roer and Henkel 1996b, p. 31f.; Wettlaufer 1996, p. 284ff., 303ff.). In Hadamar, meanwhile, the processes of increasing internal bonding and solidarity were set in motion by the organization itself: for example, employees going out to the town of Hadamar was considered fundamentally undesirable (Sandner 2003, p. 464). Even before the beginning of the gassing phase, not only offices but also numerous living, social and sleeping quarters were built and furnished for the staff (Kneuker and Steglich 1985, p. 17; Schmidt-von Blittersdorff et al. 1996, p. 82). There was great sociability among employees (Sandner 2003, p. 464; also Klee 1986, p. 128).

---

[13] "Dirty work" in its original version is related to tasks that come across as disgusting or demeaning, but above all stigmatizing (Ashforth and Kreiner 1999; Kreiner et al. 2006). Similarly, but rather reluctant to the notion of steady and high solidarity or cohesion of "dirty workers", also McCabe and Hamilton (2015).

The close-knit microculture within the murder centre, which largely excludes externalities, has the characteristics of a "social cocoon", in which norms and problem solutions created by the group or organisation itself are followed. These can develop in contrast to the rules and values represented by outsiders or even by society as a whole (Greil and Rudy 1984; also Anand et al. 2004, p. 46; Ashforth and Anand 2003, p. 9; Ermann and Lundman 1978, p. 57). Empirically this is expressed, for example, by the numerous and regular joint comradeship evenings and company outings, which – usually in the buses that were also used to transport the sick – often found their destination in other gassing facilities. All in all, the staff, according to the defendant Schmidt, "lived together in camaraderie. We were strictly barracked. We could not go out, so we sat together in the evenings after closing time" (office staff, HHStA/a, p. 120; similarly Lindner's statement, office staff, HHStA/a, p. 122f.; see also Pauline Kneissler's statement, nursing staff, Klee 1986, p. 136f.). The high degree of socialization among each other is also evident in the holidays often taken together near the institution and the many alcohol binges in nearby inns, while sexual contacts among each other were by no means the exception (Kepplinger 2008, p. 97; Klee 1986, pp. 117ff., 134, 136f.; Kneuker and Steglich 1985, p. 78ff.; Sandner 2003, p. 464; Wettlaufer 1996, p. 322ff.). The defendant Rützel was able to confirm not only the convivial drinking evenings, but many love affairs that were concluded among the staff as well (office staff, HHStA/a, p. 141).

Through the numerous joint activities of like-minded people, the employees, in addition to the other mechanisms described and many more to be described (especially Sect. 3.2), ultimately came to the conclusion that their actions cannot or could not have been so bad (Ashforth and Anand 2003, p. 14). The routines and homogeneous processes created in this context meant that potential moral difficulties associated with the actions could be removed, or at least largely suppressed (ibid., p. 12). One is immediately reminded of the statement made by nurse Paul Reuter, who only in retrospect developed a real moral awareness of his actions (Kneuker and Steglich 1985, p. 28f.). All in all, the illegal practices, it can finally be stated with regard to the pillar of institutionalization, have acquired a normative, i.e. legitimate, character with increasing time.

The process of institutionalization described previously outlines how the killings in the Hadamar asylum could be established. On the basis of certain initial social and organizational conditions on the one hand, the hierarchical-authoritarian operational structures on the other, an increasingly intensive habituation and emotional desensitization to the murderous practices developed over time, so that ethical and moral consequences could be neutralized to an advanced degree or completely faded out (Ashforth and Anand 2003, p. 13f.; Ashforth and Kreiner 2002,

p. 222f., 227f.). While the descriptions on the previous pages have primarily shown how the organized brutalities in the murder institutions could be institutionalized and stabilized as expectations of action, a rationalization of these very brutalities has remained largely absent. This problem is addressed in the following chapter.

3.2   The Rationalization of the Killings

The use of so-called "neutralization" or "rationalization strategies", "techniques" or "ideologies" generally describes the attempt of a group of actors to explain or justify deviant behavior in their profession.[14] Deviant processes (Ermann and Lundman 1978, p. 57) corresponding to valid norms and regulations are ascribed a legitimate character. They are presented as seemingly appropriate exceptions, if not as desirable practices, and in any case can, largely or even entirely, minimize the sense of guilt and responsibility of the agents for their deviations from rules. Negatively connoted interpretations of action are not only hidden in this way, but are often replaced by positive interpretations in the sense of a (specially produced) rationalization (Anand et al. 2004, p. 40f.; Bandura 1990, p. 33f.). Actors thereby convince themselves, to a certain extent, of an alleged rightness of their behaviour (Ashforth and Anand 2003, p. 15ff.; Ashforth and Kreiner 1999, p. 421ff.) and ultimately, in line with the notion of the dynamic boundaries of the zone of indifference, expand the range of what can be classified as acceptable behaviour (Adams and Balfour 2009, p. 113). To outsiders, meanwhile, these rationalizations are often met with incomprehension and appear as what they factually are: self-interested efforts to subject overtly questionable and norm-defying actions to a self-serving interpretation (Ashforth and Anand 2003, p. 17; Sykes and Matza 1957, p. 666; similarly Adams 2011, p. 277; Adams et al. 2006, p. 682). These strategies serve actors ex ante and ex post as justifying, credible and above all (self-)legitimating argumentations and perspectives with regard to a social reality that is actually to be regarded as problematic (Ashforth and Anand 2003, p. 16f.; instructive still Bandura 1990; Kaptein and van Helvoort 2018; Sykes and Matza 1957).

Since the use of these ideologies is incumbent upon the acting members of the organization themselves, this means that the techniques can be used in various intensities as well as in all kinds of combinations with one another. From an analytical point of view, this is not unproblematic: while some neutralization strategies

---

[14]There is little to no distinction made between rationalization and neutralization strategies in the literature (Kaptein and van Helvoort 2018, p. 2; see also Maruna and Copes 2005). I therefore use the terms synonymously as well.

can be quite clearly determined by various statements and positions of the Hadamar cadre, the interpretation of other statements appear more difficult and thus more ambivalent in its analytical allocation. The fundamental difficulties that arise in the use of such neutralization theories can be attributed to various circumstances – in empirical terms, for example, because some statements are simply subject to several techniques or strategies that can fluctuate over time in view of any individual variations of the staff, from a theoretical point of view, because the underlying models and heuristic (pre-)assumptions do not (or cannot) provide such unambiguous differentiation criteria at the corresponding border points (see also the more general explanations about the model in Chap. 3).

Undoubtedly, these (and certainly many more) aspects demand and promote not only the actual use, but additionally the interpretation of certain neutralization strategies or combinations instead of others. In order for the following analysis not to degenerate into a search for all kinds of different or even arbitrarily compiled techniques, I have categorized the material empirically available to me according to content and elaborated it with regard to already proven neutralization strategies (for this, see Ashforth and Anand 2003, p. 18ff.).[15] I will justify my categorizations at appropriate points, taking into account argumentative considerations regarding stringency as well as the respective focus within the statement, in order to be able to counteract possible ambiguities as far as possible. In this respect, my interpretations are not based on isolated, independent statements. Instead, I will take into account that neutralization strategies are to be located as techniques and belief systems on the group level, which enhance their credibility precisely as a result of collective use – and thus in turn also increase legitimacy for the users themselves (Ashforth and Anand 2003, p. 16; Ashforth and Kreiner 1999, pp. 419, 421; Kreiner et al. 2006, p. 619). Following this procedure, I would like to present a total of seven responsibility-relieving strategies of neutralization or rationalization in the further course of this chapter, in order to then present them on the basis of some exemplary empirical manifestations of the Hadamar asylum murders.

---

[15] There is a multitude of different neutralization or rationalization ideologies, which themselves contain manifestations of various variations and versions. Kaptein and van Helvoort (2018, p. 5f.), for example, have been able to identify 2 central strands, 4 further categories, 12 techniques, and a total of 60 associated sub-techniques in their model-like account of neutralization techniques. In this respect, I will supplement the pillar of rationalization in places with Kaptein and van Helvoort's account, but will primarily be guided by Ashforth and Anand's (2003; but further, Anand et al. 2004; Ashforth and Kreiner 1999) portrayal.

3.2.1   On the (Alleged) Legality of the Eugenic Action

A first technique for rationalizing actions is associated with legal legitimacy. Although the practiced acts are illegitimate or even illegal, actors defend and rationalize their acts with the objection that they are actually still acceptable after all because, for example, they have not been explicitly presented as wrong (Ashforth and Anand 2003, p. 18; further Kaptein and van Helvoort 2018, p. 11).

In fact, there was never any legal basis for the euthanasia campaign (Ebbinghaus 2008, pp. 214f., 223; HHStA/b, p. 30f.; Klee 1986, pp. 85ff., 302ff.; Meusch 2006, p. 311ff.). The only official document on the part of the Nazi regime was the aforementioned "euthanasia authorization" (Sect. 1.3), which served as the equivalent of a legal norm in internal circles, but was ultimately never published in legal form. On the contrary, not only the action, but even the authorization was kept secret during the Nazi era. However, it was always communicated to the staff that a legally legitimizing regulation would exist:

A: I didn't really think anything of it. I was told: this is a law from the Führer, and we have to carry out the Führer's order.

Q: (Caveat: "Führer commands, we follow" – no thoughts at all?)

A: Actually yes. That was my opinion. (statement Reuter, nursing staff, HHStA/a, p. 65)

Were the contents of the comfort letters untrue? – I did not believe I was doing anything wrong. I was told that it was the law, I believed that. I was told that by the head of the institution. (statement Schmidt, office staff, HHStA/a, p. 120)

He wanted to draw my attention to the fact that there was a law, but it had not yet been published, but it would be published after the war, according to which the seriously mentally ill and incurable people would be eliminated in a humane way. Then I got very unsettled, because I had no idea of such a thing. He said I didn't have to get upset about it at all, I had nothing to do with the sick, it was not a punishable act. (statement Gerst, office staff, HHStA/a, p. 150)

I didn't ask about the law, it was a law of the Führer for me and I was used to obedience. Inwardly I did not reproach myself. (statement by Zachow, nursing staff, quoted from Wettlaufer 1996, p. 308)

These passages may suffice for clarification. The rationalization of the deeds by an (allegedly) inherent legal basis of the events is a strategy frequently used by the Hadamar cadre (see additionally Lichtefellt, nursing staff, HHStA/a, p. 144; Siegert, office staff, HHStA/a, p. 132). In this context, the statement by clerk Gerst that an official law should be published after the war is certainly particularly interesting. Employee Lindner also pointed out that it was mentioned to him that an official law would only be promulgated after the war for reasons of secrecy as well as protection against enemy propaganda (HHStA/a, p. 122). The former T4 senior medical expert (*T4-Obergutachter*) Werner Heyde stated in the course of his hearing (HHStA/a, pp. 337 f., 341) that work was indeed being done on a foreseen legality. Corresponding drafts, which were to be made public only after the (won) war, had already existed. Similarly, Aly (1985a, p. 15f., 2013, p. 183) shows that a "law on euthanasia for the terminally ill" was drafted as early as 1940, but ultimately never published because Hitler refused to at that time (Klee 1986, p. 87ff.; Mitscherlich and Mielke 1995, p. 239ff.).

In this context, Ashforth and Anand's (2003, p. 18) assumption is confirmed, according to which particularly powerful or large organisations can make use of the possibility to create special guidelines or (organisational) laws that create a legitimising character for the actions carried out by their members. The Nazi regime or the numerous Nazi organizations with an affinity for violence are certainly idealtypical examples of this (see also Adams and Balfour 2009). The law supposedly instigated by the "Führer" could be presented to the euthanasia foot soldiers as the law that actually applied – especially since, in line with the pillar of institutionalization, one must take into account that the murders were not only legitimized by the long prehistory or initial phase as well as the historical context in general (similarly in HHStA/b, p. 30; Welzer 2005, p. 249), but also that the fundamental conception of legal law was authorized by those higher up in the hierarchy within the organization:

> Then we were led to Herr Klein and Landesrat Bernotat in Hadamar. […] Then we were taken to the Chief of Police, Mr. Bünger, who said that a law had been issued by the Führer that the incurable insane were to be killed in a humane way by gas here in Hadamar. Then he gave me a note – I can no longer say exactly what it said, but it said that I must not say a word about what had happened in Hadamar, and that I was not allowed to take any photographs, as that would be punished by death; I had to sign it. (statement by L. Thomas, nursing staff, HHStA/a, p. 58)

> Q: I ask the defendant to state whether anything was said at her introduction to Columbus House that it was the law and she was threatened with adverse consequences?

> A: Yes, there was talk of a law that existed, but that would not be published until after the war. We were reminded of the obligation to maintain secrecy and if we did not keep our mouths shut, we were threatened with concentration camps and the Gestapo. (statement by Zielke, nursing staff, HHStA/a, p. 101)[16]

---

[16] The Columbus House was the original quarters of the Central Office, i.e. before the move to Tiergartenstrasse 4 took place (Sandner 2003, p. 372).

Klein himself, in his court case after the war, answered the question of whether the employees had known about the euthanasia authorization with a yes – however, he added that the employees were always communicated an actual law. The killings of the (allegedly) terminally ill thus seemed not only legally correct (Bryant 2005, p. 82), but also to be within the employees' zone of indifference (Kühl 2014a, p. 295; Gruber and Kühl 2015, p. 20).

3.2.2 Recalibration

Several rationalization strategies can be subsumed under the purpose of shifting (Sect. 3.2.2) or transforming (3.2.3–3.2.5) the actually existing illegal and immoral character of the actions (Ashforth and Anand 2003, p. 21f.; Ashforth and Kreiner 1999, p. 421ff.). Adams and Balfour (2009, pp. 4, 9, 112) speak of a "moral inversion": here, malicious or destructive acts are subjected to positive reinterpretations, whereupon the acts are understood as no longer really bad, possibly even as good, beneficial, valuable or similar notions (see also Adams 2011; Adams et al. 2006; Reed 2012).

In the first variant of this method, "recalibration" or "refocusing," the actors do not necessarily deny the negative aspects and circumstances of their activities, but point to the supposedly positive aspects of the work, so that the objectionable features are ultimately overlooked or superimposed. In this context, salient but undesirable factors are reduced in importance, while at the same time the actually desirable but comparatively meaningless components of the event are (over-)emphasized (Ashforth and Anand 2003, p. 21f.; Ashforth and Kreiner 1999, p. 422f.; similarly Kaptein and van Helvoort 2018, p. 7f.).

As an example for Hadamar, we can refer to the cemetery caretaker Philipp Baum, who used this rationalization strategy in a conversation in two ways: While describing the beginning of his time in the asylum, he never once referred to his own (co-)participation in the murders. It seems to have escaped his notice that he was part of an organization that had carried out the mass murder of thousands of people. In any case, he expressed his incomprehension of the 30-year prison sentence because, according to his own statement, he had not been guilty of anything and had "not touched any living or dead person" (technical staff, quoted from Kneuker and Steglich 1985, p. 45). Blum, however, attributed greater importance to the two patients whose lives he had saved by referring to their ability to work, which was useful to the institution. Furthermore, Blum particularly emphasized that he had always designed the cemetery uniquely, including an extraordinary floral decoration and various wooden crosses including numbering at the graves (ibid.). Elsewhere, Sister Pauline Kneissler pointed out that the sick in the asylum – if in exceptional cases they were not or could not be taken directly to the gas chamber – were treated by the nursing staff in a very regular and caring manner until their death:

> I must expressly emphasize that the sick were treated by us, i.e., the doctors and nursing staff, as in any institution, until their death. As an example, I would like to mention that, for example, Dr. Baumhardt [doctor at Grafeneck from Jan. 1940, doctor at Hadamar from Jan. 1941-June 1941, DF] was very displeased and strongly reproached us when patients spend the night walking barefoot across the corridor to the toilet due to their mental illness – which often could not be avoided or only with difficulty (statement by Kneissler, nursing staff, quoted from Klee 1986, p. 136)

Following a similar logic, the office employee Bacher (HHStA/a, p. 148) stated that although she was aware of having given false causes of death, in her opinion it was more important to at least inform the family members at all via a letter of consolation in order not to put them into further turmoil or uncertainty.

3.2.3   Denial of Responsibility

With the technique of "denial of responsibility," there is no longer just a recalibration or refocusing, but a transformation of the actually illegal character of one's own action. In this sense, agents try to justify that they had no choice but to engage in the activities due to external factors that they consider beyond their control (Ashforth and Anand 2003, p. 18; also Ashforth and Kreiner 1999, p. 422; Sykes and Matza 1957, p. 667f.). Once again, the wrong or harmful action may in principle be acknowledged and named as such, but much or even all of the accompanying guilt is negated by reference to a reduced or complete lack of competence (Kaptein and van Helvoort 2018, p. 13; further Adams et al. 2006, p. 683; Bandura 1990, p. 36f.).

One of these reasonings was the financial dependence on the employees, which was of significant importance, especially in the case of nursing staff (Benedict and Kuhla 1999, p. 260 f.). The majority of the later accomplices learned their profession in exceedingly poor working as well as generally unstable social and economic conditions, which were caused, among other things, by Germany's recent past at the time (Benedict 2003, p. 77; Wettlaufer 1996, p. 300ff.; furthermore Hoffmann 2010, p. 253f.). This aspect can be particularly explained with regard to male employees, who had started the nursing profession in large part due to previous existing or threatening unemployment. Ultimately, however, the concern of existential insecurity is found to a high degree in both, male and female employees (Wettlaufer 1996, p. 284f., 300f., 303f.; furthermore Hoffmann 2010, p. 254). The nurses Hackbarth (Kintner 1948, p. 141) as well as Zachow (Wettlaufer 1996, p. 314), for example, have pointed out that neither of them had an own accommodation besides the existing living facilities in the Hadamar asylum. The search for other accommodation, however, was associated with problematic consequences in the context of the war (Benedict 2003, p. 77). The orderly Willig (nursing staff, Kintner 1948, p. 82) expressed that he would not have been able to leave his position simply because otherwise he would have lost his pension and would have additionally been imprisoned. For the organization, meanwhile, these ties to the institution went hand in hand with the advantage that on-site accommodation enabled further isolation and almost permanent availability of these same employees (Benedict 2003, p. 77), ultimately leading to further strengthening of the social cocoon and the group- or organization-internal rules perpetrated within it (Sect. 3.1).

Furthermore, a factor relevant in the context of denial of responsibility and recurrent in the empirical material is the repeated reference to the chain of command in the institution (Ashforth and Anand 2003, p. 18; Ashforth and Kreiner 1999, p. 422). Based on members' usual separation between their "natural person" and facets of the "organizational actor" (Balcke 2001, p. 80), one consequence of authoritarian orders is the moral exoneration of hierarchically subordinate agents (Anand et al. 2004, p. 42; Balcke 2001, p. 81; Bandura 1990, p. 34; Weissmann 2015, p. 89). It is well known that people find it easier to commit morally questionable or deviant acts if there are superiors who are prepared to take responsibility for them – or if this responsibility can at least be transferred to the higher authorities from the perspective of the subordinates (Bandura 1990, p. 34ff.; Zimbardo 2009, p. xi; see also Sect. 3.1):

> Then I said to myself again: The doctor who gives the orders as a superior bears the responsibility. Every one of the nurses during the training sessions were always told: The doctor's orders must be obeyed as a superior. If a nurse refuses to do so, or does something wrong by mistake, the nurse in question is called useless. That was about the talk of the doctors at the training sessions. And the doctor as a superior had to be obeyed. We were always commanded and it was always said that the one who gives the orders also bears the responsibility. (statement by Reuter, nursing staff, HHStA/a, p. 68f.)

The multi-level selection system, which decided on the life and death of the sick, represented an extremely potent possibility for various prison staff to relieve them from their responsibility. Accordingly, many members invoked the responsibility of higher-ranking people when reflecting on their own actions (Schmidt-von Blittersdorff et al. 1996, p. 113). As already indicated (Sect. 3.1), this was particularly true for the nursing staff in view of the doctors working in the institutions (Lilienthal 2006b, p. 286; Wettlaufer 1996, pp. 292f., 306f., 306ff.). Confirming this, Sister Pauline Kneissler claimed, "We had no responsibility, everything was done by the doctors" (nursing staff, Wettlaufer 1996, p. 308), or nurse Paul Reuter, "First of all, I did not feel responsible for the way things were done, but thought that the one who gave the order was also responsible for it. I still hold this view today" (Nurses, Wettlaufer 1996, p. 308).

Incidentally, at this point we can now identify the reason why no killings can be found away from the systematically structured plan: Since the discharge of responsibility is inherently linked to the membership in the organisation, this cognitive protective mechanism would disappear the moment that killings took place outside the organisational role. Consequently, any discharge of responsibility, at least in the present case, is bound solely to the formal role structure (Balcke 2001, p. 86; further Adams 2011, p. 276; Adams and Balfour 2009, p. 4; Bandura 1990, pp. 35, 37). Thus, the almost mechanical-looking daily routine of some staff members, who participated in exceedingly ordinary (leisure or family) activities between and after their killing routines, can also be explained (Chroust et al. 1989, pp. 112ff.). Here, sociologically speaking, one can simply observe a role change between the personal and the formal role.

3.2.4 Victim Denial

The second form of transformation, "denial of victim", allows for two central interpretations in the present case. In the first interpretation, the victims are not seen as such because they either deserved the consequences resulting from the actions or allegedly even desired them themselves (Ashforth and Anand 2003, p. 19f.; Ashforth and Kreiner 1999, p. 422; also Sykes and Matza 1957, pp. 665, 668). In the context of the euthanasia murders, this idea became established among numerous institution employees because they were convinced, apparently or in fact, that life would be a torment for the supposedly incurably ill and that death should therefore be interpreted as an act of mercy (exemplary also Lilienthal 2006b, pp. 268, 286; Sandner 2003, p. 422ff.):

> What other impression did the people in the gas chamber make on me? I was of the opinion that they were not healthy, not normal people, but actually sick people. Their hair hung in their faces, their mouths were distorted. (statement Lindner, office staff, HHStA/a, p. 126)

> Agreed with the cause? I was actually in agreement with the tasks of the action, as the doctor had explained to us, that the incurable mentally ill were killed by the euthanasia procedure; that made sense to me. Once you have seen mentally ill people, you absolutely have to say that it was the right thing to do, that they were no longer capable of living at all. [...] There were very often cripples among them and some kind of physical deformities, with thick heads or something else, where the hands had grown; you could see that. (statement Schirre, office staff, HHStA/a, p. 146)

What is striking about these and many other similar statements is that it was explicitly pointed out that it was *exclusively* a matter of very or incurably ill people, so that the killings could be presented as redemption, corresponding to euthanasia in the true sense. The above-mentioned employee Schirre, for example, emphasized again in the further course of her testimony that no curable patients were murdered in Hadamar (HHStA/a, p. 146). The assumption in this context is that this is a intensive form of (victim) denial – for there is no doubt that many sick people became victim to the eugenic campaign who could very well have carried out at least light work and thus should have been spared in accordance with the underlying euthanasia idea (see, for example, the statement by Zielke, nursing staff, HHStA/a, p. 95f.; alternatively, see also the thoughts of "estate administrator Maximilian L." – probably meaning Lindner –, who pointed out that "many of those killed may have had lucid moments", quoted after Klee 1986, p. 125). Without a doubt, this should have been noticed especially by the staff working in the care sector, who were thus directly connected to the killing processes.

The second central interpretation of victim denial can be observed – alluded to in the passage from the office worker Schirre quoted above – in connection with the dehumanization of the sick that took place at the societal as well as the organizational level. In this way, an extensive or even complete "dehumanization" of patients occurred (Weißmann 2015; further Kühl 2014a, p. 211ff.). The starting point of such dehumanization processes is a demarcation by the perpetrators, not only excluding the victims but also denying them the status of being human (Bandura 1990, p. 38; Weißmann 2015, p. 81) – as was the case years before the actual start of euthanasia in the initial period described (see Sect. 3.1). This agenda, then, was continued at the time of the gas murders:

> I had the job of undressing people. People were happy to see something different. It had been very bad human material. They were entertaining themselves in their delusions. There were many people who, apart from their mental state, had physical infirmities, who had TB, who arrived already rotten, lying in their own excrement. (statement Zielke, nursing staff, HHStA/a, p. 95 f.).

> In addition to this, the majority of the selected death candidates were ill in the body from infectious diseases, typhus, dysentery, TB. Mentally, they were also no different from an animal. (statement by Margot R.-G., nursing staff, quoted from Wettlaufer 1996, p. 309)

> In Herborn it was decidedly better. Hadamar contained the final conditions. (statement by Lückoff, nursing staff, HHStA/a, p. 99)

In view of the extremely unfavourable conditions in the asylums, many of the patients were already in such a poor physical and psychological condition on their arrival in the death camps that they seemed to confirm the propagandistically painted image of the sick (Roer and Henkel 1996b, p. 24; Wettlaufer 1996, p. 310; see also Sects. 6.1.4 and 6.2 for a continuation or intensification of this in the second murder phase).

Another practice of dehumanization, carried out almost daily in the asylum, can be observed in the markings made on the sick (Aly 2013, p. 68f.; Schmidt et al. 2012, p. 283). In this sense, the terminally ill became more of an object than a subject of the psychiatric efforts rendered by the nurses and caregivers and, in accordance with National Socialist regulations, were marked as "unworthy of life" (Aly 2013, p. 88; Klee 1986, pp. 105f., 122ff., 247ff.; Wettlaufer 1996, p. 293). Meanwhile, the exact opposite process of "humanization" is described in a survival report from the Grafeneck asylum: In this example, a marking – in this case a number affixed to the back for further bureaucratic processing of (death) cases – was removed from a supposedly sick person within a very short time. She had been classified by the investigating commission as fit for work and thus worthy of life (Aly 2013, p. 81ff.).

The certainly most bizarre example that can be found in Hadamar is based on a literally celebrated dehumanization of the sick. More precisely, this was the celebration organized by the staff – some also say: forced by the doctors or superiors (see, for example, statement Rützel, office staff, HHStA/a, p. 141; statement Schirre, office staff, HHStA/a, p. 146; statement Gerst, office staff, HHStA/a, p. 151) – which took place for the purpose of the cremation of the 10,000 corpses, including alcohol and music:

> A: I want to describe another incident that happened at the time of the cremation of the 10000th corpse. As I came down at that time, the corpse was laid out and decorated with flowers. The corpse was naked. It was lying in front of the furnace, on the stretcher. Then all the staff came down and a short speech was given. I believe that Oberlt. Bünger spoke. The whole staff was standing there. I assumed it was all the personnel. I didn't pay any attention to it. They were each given 1 bottle of beer in the burn room. I didn't think that was appropriate. I considered that a mockery.

Q: Defendant Lindner, tell us what happened.

A: In the evening after dinner a doctor said, everything must go down now, the 10000th body is being burned. The tables were in a horseshoe shape and we went down, one behind the other. When you came in, on the left, there was a stretcher, there was a dead man on it. He was covered with 24 flowers. I was one of the last to go, so I kept a low profile. Then someone appeared, I don't know if it was Merkle or Lohmann, wearing his skirt backwards and imitating a funeral by the clergy. I felt it was a mockery. I left the room because it disgusted me. He sang in a tone similar to when a mass is sung in a Catholic church. First Bünger spoke, he spoke of the action, that the law would be a benefit, that you would destroy the people who were a burden to themselves and others; that you could use the funds for other purposes, etc. (testimony Gomerski, technical Staff, and testimony Lindner, office staff, HHStA/a, p. 107)[17]

The practiced and openly expressed dehumanization of the sick can certainly be attributed a particularly high significance for the successful implementation of victim denial or rationalization in a more general sense. This can be demonstrated not only by the quantity of statements associated with it, but also by the quality: atrocities, such as (mass) killings, are demonstrably significantly easier for people to commit if they can degrade and humiliate their victims in such a way (Kühl 2014a, p. 212ff.; Weißmann 2015, pp. 79, 81ff., 123), meaning this is ultimately a highly effective technique of neutralization (Adams and Balfour 2009, p. 113). The implementation of these and numerous other dehumanization methods in the structures of the institution enabled the members to build up a consistent self-representation and to maintain it over a longer period of time (Weißmann 2015, p. 114).

3.2.5 Denial of Harm

Finally, there is another form of transformation of meaning: "denial of injury". In this context, there is no problem at all in connection with the deeds or one's own actions in the situation in question (Ashforth and Anand 2003, p. 18f.; see also Anand et al. 2004, p. 42ff.; Ashforth and Kreiner 2002, p. 218ff.; Sykes and Matza

---

[17] In accordance with the discussed difficulties concerning the forgetting and confusion of some incidents (see Sect. 1.2), it is to be pointed out for the sake of completeness that the mentioned *Lohmann* is called *Lehmann* by sister Rützel instead. Rützel confirms: "He was disguised as a clergyman and spoke in a singing tone" (HHStA/a, p. 141). However, in her opinion there was no second speaker. According to other statements, the incident occurred in the morning, after breakfast, not after dinner (see, for example, statement M. Schmidt, office staff, HHStA/a, p. 118f.; statement Schrettinger, office staff, HHStA/a, p. 138).

1957, p. 667f.). Here, the essential aspects of the previous strategies culminate together – after all, from the perspective of the euthanasia foot soldiers, one cannot be held responsible for an (alleged) harm if a genuine victim did not exist in the first place: "I did not regard the activity assigned to me as murder, but as a redemption for the sick, for in my conviction they were really incurably ill" (statement by L. Thomas, nursing staff, quoted after Lilienthal 2006b, p. 268).

It is much easier to implement this approach if the (allegedly) inflicted harm is not visible or otherwise not ascertainable (Ashforth and Anand 2003, p. 19; also Bandura 1990, p. 37; see also McCabe and Hamilton 2015, who highlight the relevance of distance-enabling technologies in such processes). Ashforth and Anand (2003, p. 19) conclude that individuals generally develop a (moral) problem with their illegal actions primarily when the suffering of others is observable (similarly Bandura 1990, p. 37). Such inhibitions to killing as well as general inhibitions in situations of violence have already been noted in numerous studies in the sociology of violence (especially in Collins 2011; summarized by Firkus 2017). In Hadamar, however, members were able to successfully avoid these difficulties because staff's actual contact with the immediate killing process was reduced to the bare minimum. Thus, although the nursing staff participated in the transports and the systematic procedures that followed, they removed themselves as soon as the sick entered the gas chamber, potentially even earlier (Wettlaufer 1996, p. 297). In fact, within the framework of the strict division of labour already mentioned (Sect. 3.1), there was never any of the emotional tension that usually occurs in confrontational situations (Collins 2009, 2011), because none of the participants had to assert themselves in such a situation in the first place:

> How far did I take the sick? I helped undress the sick and took them as far as the corridor. From there they came to the doctor, through other orderlies. From the doctor they were weighed, measured, photographed, and then they came to the cellar. We went with them only as far as the cellar stairs, we didn't need to go any further and couldn't because we always had to go back to fetch people. (statement by Reuter, nursing staff, HHStA/a, p. 65)

> My job was just to accompany the transport, show it to the doctor and then escort the patients to the bottom of the stairs. From there, there was other personnel, mostly older personnel. I did not take anyone into the gas chamber. I did not go in out of interest. I did not witness any gassing. I did not look through the window. I also did not attend a cremation. (statement by Moos, nursing staff, HHStA/a, p. 92)

> But I really had the feeling that the elimination of the sick was not my concern and was none of my business. My activities were limited to purely nursing care. (statement by Ernst Z., nursing staff, quoted from Wettlaufer 1996, p. 310)

Moreover, the final act of killing, which took place via the gas supply in the small tiled room of approx. 12.5 m² was – according to a formal regulation in the organisation – carried out solely by the doctor (Kepplinger 2008, p. 84; Sandner 2003, p. 463; Schmidt-von Blittersdorff et al. 1996, p. 91):

> What did I do when they were paraded? I went and got the next sick person and undressed them until the whole transport was processed. They were all first taken to the doctor, and afterwards there was a photo room where they were photographed, sitting, from the front, from the side and standing. [...] Then they were taken to the gas room. Involved in this? No. We only had to lead the sick to the doctor and walk to the cellar door. We didn't have to go down the stairs, the orderlies did that. Did I see the gassing process? No, never. (statement by L. Thomas, nursing staff, HHStA/a, p. 59)

Significant for the remarks about maintaining a distance to the actual killing process are also the statements of the nurses Härtle and Moos, who, in view of their accompanying role, emphasized the non-violent procedure of the transports, i.e. that at least no *unnecessary* violence was used (similar to Welzer 2005, p. 144):

> It probably happened from time to time that one or the other patient was box-legged, but actual violence or violent measures did not occur. (statement by Moos, nursing staff, HHStA/a, p. 92)

> Used force? No. [...] Whether other nurses have used violence? I saw nothing of direct violence. [...] I didn't want to say that violence was used against the patients in any way. I only wanted to say that there were sick people standing there, not moving, that they were taken and pushed away so that they could find their way back into the track. But that somehow a force would have been exercised, that I have not seen. [...] But it is not a matter of any aggressive violence, neither by me nor by anyone else, I have not noticed that. (statement by Härtle, nursing staff, HHStA/a, p. 71f.)

At the same time, the burners also had only limited involvement with the actual murder process, because their work commitment only began after the gas chamber had been aired out. The sick were already dead by this time. This task was generally perceived as the worst and, especially from a psychological point of view, the most exhausting. But inhibitions in the face of possible face-to-face confrontations could not arise here either. Accordingly, it is not surprising that the burners, who after all were still most likely to be confronted with the immediate death of the people, were generally not supposed to have any previous direct contact – unlike the (accompanying) nursing staff – with the later victims (Lilienthal 2006b, p. 283). On the contrary, a far-reaching rule for the burners was to avoid any contact: "When it was said that a transport was coming, our group, if it was on duty, went down and heated the two ovens" (Klee 1986, p. 124; see also 126f.).[18]

3.2.6   For the Benefit of the Higher Purpose

A supportive rationalization refers to a supposedly higher determination of actions that goes beyond universalistic norms (Ashforth and Anand 2003, p. 21). In the case of euthanasia, we can first point to internal solidarity, which was characterized by a "climate of demanding loyalty" (Lilienthal 2006b, p. 288; see also Wettlaufer 1996, p. 313f.). Thus, a necessary criterion within the foster care was the consideration of the norms of comradeship, which was already pointed out in the training (ibid., p. 292), but also in the Hadamar institution itself (Sandner 2003, p. 286).[19]

Much more generally, the killings can be interpreted in terms of or for the benefit of a higher purpose, according to which the hereditary health policy implemented in practice was intended to serve the overarching National Socialist social plan, the Volksgemeinschaft, which hovered over all socially educated people and individualities (Schmuhl 2011a, p. 25; Wettlaufer 1996, p. 292; instructive also Schmuhl 2008).[20] Once again, the significance of the individual was defined in terms of his or her value to society. In the context of eugenic operation, such rationalistic calculations can be found in the training of nursing staff, as the following excerpt from a central textbook of nursing instruction published in 1939 shows:

---

[18] Elsewhere Lilienthal (2006a, p. 160) writes that the sick were led from the burners into the shower room. However, all other sources – including Lilienthal himself – point out that this was not the case. This refers to reports from other asylums (Klee 1986, pp. 124, 127) as well as to those from Hadamar (Lilienthal 2006b, pp. 283, 285; Schmidt-von Blittersdorff et al. 1996, p. 90f.; Wettlaufer 1996, p. 297), which is why no further attention is paid to this version.

[19] Camaraderie refers to a particularly far-reaching form of collegiality. Expectations of camaraderie among hierarchical equals are exacerbated by pressure from those of higher rank (Kühl 2017b).

[20] The extent to which the social model of the Volksgemeinschaft was a myth or reality is disputed in research. However, it is quite clear that the formula of the Volksgemeinschaft, which the Nazi regime liked to use for propaganda purposes, at least had a certain social thrust and mobilising power (Bajohr and Wildt 2009), as can also be seen in the present case. Its importance lies within these implications. Whether the Volksgemeinschaft represented an *actual* social state is neither to be asserted nor excluded (ibid.). In fact, it is of no further importance in this context whether the topos of the Volksgemeinschaft was based on real or "fictitious consensus" (Luhmann 1995, p. 68f.; see also Kühl 2014a, p. 97ff.).

> A positive attitude towards the National Socialist state is a matter of course, if only for the reason that the nurse would otherwise not be able to understand the basic laws of life, which form the pillars of the National Socialist world view and also play an infinitely important role in the professional circle of the nurse. […] it is the general public that has to pay for the needs of the sanatoriums and nursing homes with its taxes. But the good of the people must be even more sacred than one's own possessions. (Faltlhauser 1939, quoted after Wettlaufer 1996, p. 292)

It should be emphasized in this context that professional nurse training had already been a significant indoctrination tool in many respects since 1933, given its teaching premises were in line with the National Socialist social and world view (Jütte 2011, p. 97). In this racial-ideological paradigm, the respective nurses no longer found themselves in the usual role of supporting the sick and those in need of help, but instead functioned as enforcers of socially necessary sanctions against the allegedly unfit in order to contribute to the "optimization of the 'body of the people'" (Schmuhl 2011c, p. 215; see also Hoffmann 2010, p. 255; Sandner 2003, pp. 238f., 370, 481; Wettlaufer 1996, p. 292ff.).

There is no doubt that the practices ultimately carried out may have been recognized as a (necessary) evil, as has already been suggested in the context of some previous rationalization strategies. But in most cases, the end was quite capable of legitimizing the means employed, and thus of rationalizing the action, if necessary, even on a more comprehensive level (for this also Adams and Balfour 2009, p. 9f.; Katz 1993, p. 25; Perrow 2009, p. xixf.). Thus, although the killings were perhaps not always approved of by all or even many members of the staff because of their form, at least the matter as a whole could be understood as indispensable or unavoidable:

> At first we did not think about our activities at Grafeneck, since we considered the elimination of truly incurable mental patients to be understandable. (statement by Zielke, nursing staff, quoted from Wettlaufer 1996, p. 309f.)

> The gassing had a deterrent effect on us, although everyone knew that death by gassing did not hurt. […] I suffered from the fact that the action went too far, and I also told the doctors. […] In 1940 I had already been working for a sanatorium and nursing home for 15 years and had become acquainted with all types of mental patients there. In my daily dealings with them I had come to the honest conviction that life no longer meant anything to many of them and that death was a salvation for them. I therefore never had the feeling that I had anything to reproach myself for when I made myself available for the execution of the euthanasia action. If I nevertheless repeatedly asked to be released after the end of the action in Hadamar, it was because our work was wearing on my nerves and I absolutely had to get out. (statement by Kneissler, nursing staff, quoted by Wettlaufer 1996, p. 319)

It is undoubted that this is associated with a continued moral inversion, i.e. that there are certainly overlaps and, above all, reinforcing effects with other rationalization strategies that set the shift (Sect. 3.2.2) or transformation (3.2.3–3.2.5) of the illegal character of the acts in motion. In particular, relieving the sick of their alleged physical and/or psychological suffering is a regularly recurring complex in the empirical material.

3.2.7   Euphemistic Vocabulary

Finally, the rationalization strategies described on the previous pages were also promoted and consolidated by the use of a very specific use of language in order to dampen possible difficulties in the thought patterns of the illegally acting actors from the outset. In this context, Bandura (1990, p. 31f.) speaks of "euphemistic labeling" in order to mask activities that are actually reprehensible in the light of a glossed-over linguistic jargon or to give them a respectable status beyond that (similarly Adams and Balfour 2009, p. 18). While this does not automatically transform the meaning of the practices, they at least convey such an impression in their linguistic communication: "Through the power of hygienic words, even killing a human being loses much of its repugnancy. [...] murder is transformed by admirable words into the honorable discharge of duty" (Bandura 1990, p. 31). For National Socialism, quite generally speaking, countless examples for the use of euphemistic vocabulary can be found (e.g. Adams and Balfour 2009, pp. 18, 114; Welzer 2005, p. 119).

For the present object of investigation, it can be pointed out that, for example, the term "murder of the sick" was rarely used. Instead, "euthanasia", being in line with the (allegedly) official goals of the campaign, namely to mercifull kill the incurable ill, provided a rather positively connotated apparatus. In written communication, Nazi personnel often resorted to the terminology of *disinfection*. To *disinfect* a sick person meant to subject him or her to gassing (see, for example, Hinz-Wessels et al. 2005, pp. 87f., 96, 107).[21] Another example can be seen upon taking a look at the murder of children as part of the T4 campaign, with terms such

---

[21] Particularly alarming in this context is the fact that in some cases, the request of a relative to send the estate of the deceased (i.e. gassed) family member was met by the killing centre – in this case Hartheim – with a reply explaining the objects in question had "suffered so much as a result of the *disinfection* that had become necessary" (quoted from Hinz-Wessels et al. 2005, p. 83f., emphasis DF) that they had been "transferred to the National Socialist People's Welfare Organisation" (ibid.).

as *therapy* or *treatment* being used in these contexts (Aly 2013, p. 35; Klee 1986, p. 238; Sandner 2003, p. 532f.).[22] By using such terminology, those involved were able to carry out other rationalization strategies, in particular victim and damage denial (Sects. 3.2.4–3.2.5), more unproblematically.

Through the numerous mechanisms described in this section, institutional staff were given the illusion of morality in their activities (Ashforth and Anand 2003, p. 23). It is clear from the reports and testimonies that staff believed their actions were in no way unlawful or morally supremely unethical. Rather, as the findings can be subsumed in a concluding sentence, a contrary position developed, according to which the actions were ascribed an exceedingly positive, often even desirable character (see also Adams and Balfour 2009, p. 17; Adams et al. 2006, p. 682f.).

3.3   The Socialization of the Killings

The rationalization strategies discussed in the previous chapter serve in principle all members of the organization, but especially new ones to be able to establish justifications and positive interpretations of illegal actions. In general, it must be assumed that "newcomers" in particular feel insecure and anxious as part of their initial experience (Anand et al. 2004, p. 44). However, strategies of socialization help to appropriately utilize or exploit the rationalization ideologies so that new organizational members can also engage in the illegal practices and legitimize them for themselves (see also Ermann and Lundman 1978, p. 58).

Since the illegal requirements in the case study examined here – i.e. the murders of the sick – were a decidedly important part of the conditions of membership, individuals who could largely identify with the internal purposes and goals of the action were primarily used for their implementation. In fact, any personnel recruitment carried out in Hadamar was based, in addition to a certain minimum level of professional suitability for the respective position, on the political loyalty or reliability of the person on the one hand, and a positive attitude towards eugenically justified mercy killing on the other (Lilienthal 2006b, pp. 269, 288; Sandner 2003, pp. 142ff., 419ff., 431f., 440; Wettlaufer 1996, pp. 295f). Sadistic personality structures or character traits, meanwhile, played no role in the admission of new

---

[22] This brief excerpt may suffice at this point. There are undoubtedly many more examples to be found – one only needs to take a closer look at the statements made by the staff so far and those that will follow in the further course of the work.

members (Wettlaufer 1996, p. 297; also Hoffmann 2010, p. 254f.; Sandner 2003, p. 428).

The successful implementation of illegal practices is additionally aided by the recruitment of employees on the basis of personal or social networks, for example through recommendations from other employees or relatives (Ashforth and Anand 2003, p. 25; Ashforth and Kreiner 1999, p. 419f.). Recruitment activities in Hadamar proceeded along the same lines: For example, the cemetery gardener and telephone operator, Philipp Blum, was the cousin of the provincial secretary and later administrative director, Alfons Klein (Kneuker and Steglich 1985, p. 41ff.), while Sister Irmgard Huber was Klein's mistress (Wettlaufer 1996, pp. 323f.). In general, it is striking in this context that a large proportion of the individuals who had already worked for the Hadamar LHA prior to the state takeover continued to be employed by the T4 organization, while at the same time individuals classified as politically unsafe or disloyal were weeded out by Klein and Bernotat (Sandner 2003, pp. 426f., 440; Wettlaufer 1996, p. 296f.). To all appearances, Klein in particular served as a comparatively reliable source of personnel selection in this context, because he had been a member of the NSDAP since 1930 and had also been active in Hadamar almost continuously since 1934 and had thus built up a corresponding network (Wettlaufer 1996, p. 296f.).

Far from this Hadamar grouping, which was already largely known, the acquisition of further employees took place in close cooperation between the T4 Central Office in Berlin and numerous supporting authorities or institutions. In addition to the political loyalty described above and the identification with the purpose of the action, the factor of internal familiarity was obligatory: almost all new recruitments had in common that they were made via recommendations from party circles, reliable contacts and/or from already active T4 staff (Lilienthal 2006b, p. 269; Sandner 2003, pp. 420, 423, 440f.; Wettlaufer 1996, p. 295f.). Alternatively, they were familiar in another sense. Such was the case for the later estate administrator Lindner, who was known due to his long party career (Sandner 2003, pp. 424ff., 440f.). The Nassau District Association, the Frankfurt Gauleitung (via the employment office) or corresponding recommendations and transfers from other state sanatoria proved to be particularly helpful here (Sandner 2003, p. 419ff.; similarly for other T4 institutions, see Hoffmann 2010, pp. 255, 257).

The Berlin staff (see Sect. 2.1), who were able to gain extensive knowledge due to their involvement in the murders of the sick at the Grafeneck killing facility, should also be mentioned in this context. They were transferred to the Hadamar LHA only after the killings in Grafeneck were concluded near the end of 1940 (Sandner 2003, p. 440; Wettlaufer 1996, p. 295). Such earlier experiences, in the context of which an initial socialization with the same or at least similar facts could already take place, usually contribute to the institutionalization and rationalization of members' actions (Anand et al. 2004, p. 39; Ashforth and Anand 2003, p. 25; also Kühl 2020a, p. 113ff.). The Hadamar killing squad was thus composed from the outset of a relatively homogeneous, a quasi (pre-)socialized group, which is why the implementation of rationalization and socialization techniques within the institution posed comparatively few problems.

In most cases, the actual strategies of socialization occur in connection with selected rationalization techniques. A first form of practiced or induced socialization took place via deliberately placed rewards, which were intended to induce employees to adjust their attitudes and behaviors in accordance with the illegal practices, because the gratifications could only be achieved if the acts were performed appropriately (Anand et al. 2004, p. 44; Ashforth and Anand 2003, p. 28f.; Campbell and Göritz 2014, p. 291f.). As an example of this, we only need to refer to the loyalty or silence bonus, which was issued not just in view of satisfactory work already done but also with a view to continued cooperation. One such document states:

> I would like to take this opportunity to thank you for your loyal cooperation and to express the hope that you will continue to place your labour fully at the disposal of the Foundation in the coming year. The amount of your credit is to be kept secret from your fellow workers. (quoted from Klee 1986, p. 130)[23]

A second socialization technique lies in a process-like introduction of the employees to the tasks. In this sense, new members in particular receive only those instructions at the beginning of their employment that correspond to a relatively small deviation from the rules. However, as time passes, expectations are raised accordingly (Anand et al. 2004, p. 45; Ashforth and Anand 2003, p. 29f.; Campbell and Göritz 2014, pp. 291f., 296). This was reported, for example, by the employee Hubert Gomerski, who initially only worked in the office at Hartheim before he had to help out at the incinerators – initially only to shovel coke. A short time later, however, he was required to participate in the actual burning of the corpses. When he was then transferred to Hadamar, he also worked in the workshop before he was again employed as a burner (Lilienthal 2006b, p. 283f.). In a similar vein, Sister Pauline Kneissler stated that the nursing staff at Grafeneck were initially occupied with household chores before "the first patients were brought in" (Kneuker and

---

[23] The mentioned "Foundation" refers to the "Charitable Foundation for Institutional Care" (*Gemeinnützige Stiftung für Anstaltspflege*), one of T4's several cover names or organizations (see, for example, Friedlander 1997, p. 134; Hinz-Wessels et al. 2005, p. 83, FN 13). Other incentives were also mentioned in Sect. 3.1.

Steglich 1985, p. 90). At first, however, only the male nurses were employed for this purpose, in order to "gradually, as we became familiar with it" (ibid.), make use of the female staff as well.

Finally, a last socializing strand lies in the loyalty obligation by the staff (Ashforth and Anand 2003, p. 31f.). Thus, the office staff was almost entirely obligated to serve in the context of the euthanasia campaign and consisted to a substantial extent of young women between 17 and 19 years (HHStA/b, p. 24ff.; further Sandner 2003, p. 423f.). Not fulfilling this obligation resulted in a severe punishment – or at least this was threatened regularly and in a credible manner (testimony Walter, employment agent, HHStA/a, p. 299ff.; for the lack of exit options in general, see also Sect. 6.1.6).[24] The Berlin personnel, when they originally began their service at the end of 1939 in Grafeneck, were also obliged to serve via the Central Office (Sandner 2003, p. 421f.; Wettlaufer 1996, p. 296f.). Similarly, it was taken care of maintaining a certain degree of voluntariness and conviction in the deployment in order to prevent too much resistance in the first place (Sandner 2003, p. 420). In addition, every member of the institution was bound to secrecy under the most severe threats of punishment, sometimes verbally or by handshake, alternatively in writing or even by both forms, in many cases multiple times during their involvement (for a list see HHStA/b, p. 33; summarizing Sandner 2003, p. 438f.; confirmation in the statements of Härtle, nursing staff, HHStA/a, p. 70; Huber, nursing staff, HHStA/a, p. 48; L. Thomas, nursing staff, HHStA/a, p. 58; Lückoff, nursing staff, HHStA/a, p. 99; Reuter, nursing staff, HHStA/a, p. 64).

Overall, the illegal practices took on an increasingly legitimate character under all of the aforementioned circumstances (Campbell and Göritz 2014, p. 294). In view of the fact that the actions were part of the institution's internal routine and that they were also carried out and instructed by the older employees or hierarchically higher superiors, new employees in particular may have come to the conclusion that the actions could not be wrong in principle, which is why they could and should be carried out without any problem (Ashforth and Anand 2003, p. 27). The

---

[24] It cannot be conclusively clarified why they were such conspicuously young women: "The girls were also much too young. I had reservations about them going to Berlin of all places. [...] No, it was *precisely* these girls who were used" (testimony Walter, employment agent, HHStA/a, p. 301, emphasis DF). The employment agent in charge at the time testified at the Frankfurt trial that she investigated this question herself because there were no obvious reasons why these and not other women or men were recruited. Ultimately, it was communicated that these women "were chosen by the department, I would not have to talk about it at all, but I would have to oblige them to serve" (ibid., p. 299). It can be assumed that the members who were obligated to serve were not chosen randomly or without reason (Sandner 2003, p. 420).

large in-group bond as well as solidarity that existed in Hadamar, including the associated camaraderie among each other, indicate at least such homogeneity of the group in this respect. Taking into consideration the numerous processes and mechanisms described, the socialization of the (new) members was a comparatively easy undertaking, because in view of the extremely careful recruitment of personnel, only potentially suitable candidates were considered anyway.

3.4 Critical Reflection: Interdependencies and Empirically Based Queries

Numerous interdependencies and entanglements have become clear in the argumentative three-step process presented. The analysis of the first murder phase has shown that not only do the three central pillars of the model influence and reinforce each other, but that very similar effects occur within the pillars themselves. It is obvious, for example, that the shifting or transformation techniques (Sect. 3.2.2–3.2.5) have fluid boundaries, while at the same time both, the higher purpose of the action (Sect. 3.2.6) and the euphemistic vocabulary used (Sect. 3.2.7), have an influence on the legitimacy of all rationalization strategies. The fact that some explanations and processes in this framework can be contradictory to each other is neither surprising nor contrary to general reasoning (Ashforth and Kreiner 1999, p. 422). Such an occurrence can be seen, for example, in the case of the nurse Lydia Thomas, who presented her (co-)participation in court with two (seemingly) contradictory arguments: on the one hand, she had genuinely wanted to help incurably ill people with mercy killing from the outset – which is equivalent to the variant of victim denial – but her actions were also a consequence of the fear of being sanctioned by someone hierarchically higher if she did not follow the instructions, which is precisely equivalent to the denial of any personal responsibility (Lilienthal 2006b, p. 286).

Enmeshments can also be observed between the pillars. In view of the conditions prevailing in the institutions, which can be understood as a consequence of the austerity policy initiated in the institutionalization, many sick people came close to such a physically poor condition that it was obviously not too difficult for the members to make use of the rationalization strategy of victim denial. In this, the process of dehumanization effectively reinforced itself (Weißmann 2015, p. 81). Likewise, it seems immediately plausible that the socialization of (new) members is not only directly linked to rationalization strategies, but that these two processes in turn also jointly contribute to the (long-)lasting institutionalization of illegality. After all, the latter can only be maintained if the participants involved do not feel compelled to question the established practices or even openly reject them – which is precisely what is prevented by the rationalization as well as socialization of the acts (Ashforth and Anand 2003, p. 35).[25]

In view of these (and many other) interdependencies, one might ask whether this should be interpreted as a strength or weakness of the conception: Are the overlaps to be interpreted in the sense that the theorem of the normalization of illegal practices allows empirical phenomena to be precisely addressed and interpreted, or are such entanglements rather the consequence of a conception that remains vague? The answer seems, to put it simply, to lie somewhere in the middle. Or, to phrase it differently – the reader may forgive my evasion to the now probably favourite answer of many sociologists –, it is above all case-dependent. Although a theoretically oriented critique might denounce the too broad views of Ashforth and Anand (2003) – respectively of the publications closely related to it (Anand et al. 2004; Ashforth and Kreiner 1999; furthermore Ashforth and Kreiner 2002) –, such an objection seems inappropriate after the evaluation of the empirical material on the past pages. The argumentative three-step approach pursued has made it clear how the National Socialist murders of the sick were institutionalized, rationalized, and socialized, and how the acts were thus ultimately normalized, i.e., they were seen as (more or less) self-evident and could be continued over a longer period of time in an almost everyday and regulated manner.

What is to be criticized, meanwhile, is the inability of many of the authors used here (such as Ashforth and Anand 2003; Brief et al. 2001; Kaptein and van Helvoort 2018) to recognize that rule deviations cannot unfold only in a kind of organizational underlife. Illegal practices do not necessarily develop and reproduce within a bounded "local rationality" (Luhmann 1995, pp. 82f., 306f.) or in a virus-like infection of the organization (Ashforth et al. 2008, p. 671), but may well be obligatory or even a mandatory behavioral expectation from the outset, as was the case in Hadamar. Such a "blind spot" can be found in numerous studies in organizational sociology or theories that refer to illegal practices in general. In many cases, to further stress this problem, no distinction is made between illegality that is useful for one's own sake and such illegality that is useful for the organization. Neither is an effort made to adopt a perspective that looks at the fulfillment of organizational

---

[25] The brief forms of interdependencies should suffice here. Many more have been at least hinted at via the analysis, and some additional ones could easily be enumerated. At this point, it is not so much of interest to list as many of these entanglements as possible, but rather to draw attention to the fact *that* many strategies and methods stand in numerous relations to one another.

purposes through the deliberate and continual use of deviations from rules or even legal rights (Luhmann 1995, p. 304ff.; see also Kühl 2020a).[26]

Finally, it can be critically questioned whether a third socialization strategy identified by Ashforth and Anand (2003, p. 30f.), which was omitted from the previous analysis, can be observed in Hadamar. This method describes a behaviour in which the actors resort to illegal practices in order to solve impending problems or conflicts. In doing so, the acts are often carried out under – at least originally – good intentions. For large parts of the nurses, it could certainly be pointed out in this context that one wanted to spare the sick the alleged tortures and accordingly help them with mercy killings (exemplarily Lilienthal 2006b, p. 285ff.). Analytically, however, the problem at this point lies in the fact that, according to this method of socialization, the actors try to help themselves with a practice that deviates from the rules, in which there would certainly be options that conform to the rules, but the actors do not hold out any prospect of success for them. However, what a realistic alternative would have looked like in a killing centre whose sole aim and purpose was the mass murder of the sick and its concealment, especially in view of the loyalty obligations (Sect. 3.3), remains an open question that possibly cannot even be answered (see also Sect. 6.1.6).

---

[26] It is noticeable, especially in many US-American debates about illegal actions in organizations, that no functionality of any kind is or can be attributed to them. Instead, it is emphasized that rule deviations have fundamentally negative effects on individuals, organizations, *and* large parts of society (for example, see Brief et al. 2001, p. 472). This is evidently clear from the comparatively limited repertoire of terms used in these surroundings, insofar as many of such papers speak explicitly of *corrupt* practices and corrupt practices only. In other words, they focus on a term that is associated from the outset with a purely negative and dysfunctional meaning: "First, corruption is a strong, provocative term. It calls attention to undesirable behavior [...]" (Ashforth et al. 2008, p. 671). This shortcoming is possibly related to the fact that deviations from rules become prominent in the public eye as soon as they are uncovered by media outlets in the course of highly stylized organizational failures (Kühl 2020a, p. 12). Nevertheless, taking into account a cost-benefit calculus from the perspective of the organization, an illegal handling of certain matters may very well be a decision made on a rational basis with numerous resulting benefits and profits – a perspective that is largely lost in such elaborations. Organizations may therefore resort to (in-)conspicuous rule deviations more or less often. They are, however, for understandable reasons, not so readily presented to the general public (ibid., pp. 11 ff., 127; also Ermann and Lundman 1978, pp. 62, 64; Luhmann 1995, p. 114f.; examples of this include the Siemens corruption case, Bergmann 2013; the rationalization tendencies at Ford, Gioia 1992; a series of short empirical case sketches of norm deviations in Culjak 2015, p. 8ff.; a classic sociological piece of literature is found in Bensman and Gerver 1963).

The (Temporary) Stop of Aktion T4

4

Presumably on August 21, 1941, Hitler gives Karl Brandt, one of the two original euthanasia authorizers (Sect. 1.3), the verbal order to stop the eugenic murders in a personal conversation. A short time later, on August 24, 1941, the euthanasia came to its (provisional) conclusion. It seems that the institutions were informed in writing (Faulstich 1998, p. 271). In Hadamar, the gas murder phase thus ends after 8 months (Klee 1986, p. 221; Lilienthal 2006a, p. 168; Schmuhl 2011c, p. 229). About 10,000 of the more than 70,200 victims were gassed in Hadamar alone (Klee 1986, p. 232). The halt hits the T4 headquarters suddenly, virtually in the midst of ongoing operations (Lilienthal 2006b, p. 270; Schmuhl 2011c, p. 229f.; Süß 2003, p. 314). Still on September 24, patients arrive at two intermediate institutions of Hadamar, Eichberg and Weilmünster (Lilienthal 2010, p. 101).

The background for the interruption of the campaign was unclear for a long time. To this day, it seems hardly possible to determine *the* crucial variable (Klee 1986, p. 221; Schmuhl 2011c, p. 221). But at least some central events can be highlighted that probably contributed to Hitler's final decision. First of all, without doubt, the reaction of the Bishop of Münster, Clemens August Graf von Galen, played a key role. In contrast to what had been presented shortly before, in a rather vaguely worded pastoraly letter of the Catholic Church in July 1941, von Galen spoke openly for the first time in three sermons about the fact that proactive mass murder of mentally and psychologically ill people was being practiced in Germany (Aly 2013, p. 175ff.; Faulstich 1998, p. 276ff.; Klee 1986, p. 193ff.; Sandner 2003, p. 503).

Even before the action was called off, the murder of the sick, originally still conceived as a secret Reich matter, resembled a rather open secret (Sandner 2003, pp. 488, 492ff.; Schmuhl 2011c, p. 229; see also the statement by Dietrich Allers, managing director of the Central Office, in Klee 1986, p. 140f.). Especially in the vicinity of the death institutions, the operation could not be concealed for long (Faulstich 1998, p. 275; Meusch 2006, p. 311f.; Stöckle 2010). In Hadamar, for example, people were struck by the permanently smoking chimney of the crematorium and the smell of burnt corpses that permeated large parts of the village (Mitscherlich and Mielke 1995, pp. 254, 256; Schmidt-von Blittersdorff et al. 1996, p. 120; similar descriptions in Grafeneck and Pirna, see Stöckle 2010, p. 120f.). Others reported how even children shouted that the "Berlin murder cart" (quoted from Sandner 2003, p. 496f.) was back when the famous transport buses arrived (see also Faulstich 1998, p. 275ff.; Mitscherlich and Mielke 1995, p. 256f.). The significance of von Galen's open rally was thus not to reveal a state secret, but to publicly address and condemn the murders, which had been largely ignored and/ or denied by the population, in order to install an awareness of their illegitimacy in the first place (Aly 2013, p. 175; Klee 1986, p. 193; also Stöckle 2010, pp. 121f.).

For the Nazi regime, these declarations were conceivably unfavorable, because at the time of von Galen's particularly significant third sermon, the German troops were encountering increased, unexpected difficulties in the war against the Soviet Union in August 1941 (Aly 2013, pp. 174, 176f.; Süß 2003, p. 316). The general low mood among the population (for this Faulstich 1998, p. 283; Kepplinger 2008, p. 100) also seemed to intensify against the backdrop of the now increasingly loud expressions of discontent and uncertainty about the eugenic campaign – although this still led to isolated protests at most (Klee 1986, p. 226ff.; Sandner 2003, p. 501; Stöckle 2010, pp. 118, 121). In any case, according to the internal opinion of some Nazi elites, one could not afford additional insecurities in the interior of the country (Sandner 2003, p. 505). Joseph Goebbels, as Reich Minister for Popular Enlightenment and Propaganda being one of the central men in the Nazi state, noted in a diary entry that one had to "avoid open conflict" (quoted from Aly 2013, p. 184) because there was a "lack of sufficient time and nerve" (ibid.) to afford additional losses of confidence or unrest among the population. Ultimately, it was precisely for these reasons that the regime did not take action against von Galen (Faulstich 1998, p. 280ff.; Friedlander 1997, p. 198; Sandner 2003, p. 503).

At this time, however, foreign countries were already informed about the eugenic campaign (Faulstich 1998, p. 278f.). After the events had already been reported in foreign media since the beginning of 1941, the British Air Force increasingly dropped leaflets in large German cities from June onwards, in which the murders of the sick and disabled were discussed, further rumours were spread and, among other things, the third sermon by von Galen was printed (Kepplinger 2008, p. 100; Sandner 2003, pp. 496, 500). Thereupon, primarily due to the outlined domestic as well as foreign policy reasons, it came to the demonstrative stop of the action. Meanwhile, the thesis that the sick killings were stopped because the planned target of 70,000 deaths (which had been raised several times in the meantime) had been reached or exceeded by 273 can be rejected for empirically comprehensible reasons (for this, see Aly 2013, p. 44ff.; Faulstich 1998, p. 272ff.; Sandner 2003, p. 504f.; Schmuhl 2011c, p. 229f.). The interruption of the action is primarily to be interpreted as a reaction with regard to the political as well as military events (Aly 2013, p. 174).

4.1 After the Stop: Alternative Activities of the Personnel

For several decades, the myth persisted that after the euthanasia halt described above, there was actually a definitive cessation of the campaign (Sandner 2003, p. 506). In fact, the opposite happened: although it was not certain, or could not be certain, whether and how things would continue (see, for example, Lilienthal 2010, p. 101; Schmidt-von Blittersdorff et al. 1996, p. 99; Süß 2003, p. 314), no one was dismissed by the Central Office; some employees probably did not even notice that there had been an interruption at all (Klee 1986, pp. 221f., 259). Instead, the action was now given a legally legitimate form: by decree, the newly created institution of the "Reich Commissioner for the Sanatoria and Nursing Homes" was established in October 1941. Two months after the termination of the operation, an official institution for the murders of the sick was thus created by the Nazi government (Aly 1985a, p. 16f., 2013, p. 47, 184ff.; Chroust et al. 1989, p. 66; Sandner 2003, p. 511). In terms of personnel, a certain Dr. Herbert Linden was designated for this purpose – an important figure, especially in the second phase of the euthanasia action (see Chap. 5), who remains surprisingly undescribed in the related literature (Aly 2013, p. 185; Faulstich 1998, p. 293f.).

In addition, a few weeks after the demonstrative halt, a meeting was held in Schloss Sonnenstein, which until then had functioned as a gassing facility, at which senior T4 officials informed the staff members, seconded from all the institutions on 27 or 28 November 1941, that the operation had not ended, but would continue promptly, or at the latest after the end of the war (Klee 1986, p. 283; Lilienthal 2010, p. 101; Sandner 2003, pp. 506, 522f.). For the Central Office, the task in this interim period was therefore to maintain its personnel potential, which was widely distributed throughout the Reich, and to find them alternative areas of responsibility (Süß 2003, p. 314f.). For this purpose, the employees of T4 or the respective institutions were initially kept on. Thus, the employees from Hadamar remained active in their institution. Some were assigned to cleaning work (Lilienthal 2010,

p. 101; statement L. Thomas, nursing staff, HHStA/a, p. 59). The office staff continued to work on administrative tasks that had been left undone until then (statement Schmidt, office staff, HHStA/a, p. 118; statement Schirre, office staff, HHStA/a, p. 146) and, in particular, dealt with the processing of the eugenic action at Grafeneck in the course of the "Abwicklungsabteilung Grafeneck" (winding-up department Grafeneck) (Friedlander 1997, p. 162f.). The aim was to bring the murder of the sick to a bureaucratic conclusion and thus to prepare accordingly for the action that might be continued in the future (Sandner 1999, p. 389f.). In June or July 1942, all files (which by then had probably been processed to the greatest possible extent) were then transported by truck to Berlin (Lilienthal 2006b, p. 270; Sandner 1999, p. 394, 2003, p. 523f.). Beyond that, however, there was a lack of concrete tasks for the rest of the Hadamar cadre. Some of them were therefore ordered to the district institutions Eichberg and Weilmünster in the period from December 1941 to about June 1942 (Sandner 2003, p. 523ff.; Wettlaufer 1996, p. 298f.).

At the same time, large parts of the T4 personnel, including some hitherto under-exposed forces from Hadamarer, were used in the context of other orders (Friedlander 1997, p. 228ff.; Lilienthal 2006b, p. 270f.). In Germany itself, this included the "Aktion" or "Sonderbehandlung 14f13," in which at least 20,000 concentration camp prisoners were murdered in the gas chambers of the T4 institutions at Bernburg, Hartheim, and possibly Sonnenstein (for this, see Sandner 2003, p. 504) – which means that the gassings at this time were only actually stopped in Hadamar (Aly 2013, p. 48f.; Hinz-Wessels et al. 2005, p. 88f.; Kepplinger 2008, p. 93f.; Schmuhl 2011c, p. 230).[1] Outside Germany, the focus was, among other things, on the shrouded-in-secrecy "Osteinsatz," in which some of the T4 personnel were deployed in the depths of wartime winter between January and March 1942 under the direction of Viktor Brack in what was Belarus at the time to (allegedly)

---

[1] It therefore does not seem unreasonable to interpret National Socialist euthanasia, as it had been practiced up to that point, as a kind of catalyst that also (co-)influenced the Holocaust in one way or another (Schmuhl 2011c, p. 214f.; for more details, see Friedlander 1997). It may be inappropriate to speak of a (proactive "test run", because one would have to implicitly assume that the Holocaust was a crime that had always been planned and structured, but this is certainly disputed (see, for example, Broszat 1977; Browning 1989). Nevertheless, it is of course striking that not only for "Aktion 13f14", but also for the external undertakings (still to follow in the main text), such as "Aktion Reinhardt", many of the "gassing specialists" (Broszat 1977, p. 747) known from euthanasia were employed. It is not improbable that, at relatively short notice but probably quite consciously, recourse was made to already existing empirical values in theory and practice (see also Browning 1989, pp. 202, 204; Sandner 2003, p. 528).

rescue and assist wounded soldiers (Browning 1989, p. 204; Kepplinger 2008, p. 102f.; Sandner 2003, p. 526f.). According to Sandner (2003, p. 526f.), more than 30 T4 employees took part in the Eastern mission, more than 20 of whom had previously been employed in Hadamar, while Schmidt-von Blittersdorff et al. (1996, p. 99) assume that up to 40 Hadamar employees were involved. It has never been definitively clarified why the details of the operation were also kept secret internally (for this, for example, see Chroust et al. 1989, p. 61; Sandner 2003, p. 526). Inevitably, this raises the question of whether T4 personnel on the war front "euthanized" sick or seriously injured soldiers (Kepplinger 2008, p. 102f.; Schmidt-von Blittersdorff et al. 1996, p. 100). The nurse Pauline Kneissler, who worked in Hadamar from the end of 1940 (Sandner 2003, p. 733), for example, has provided a statement according to which she would have greatly regretted "having given injections in the military hospital in Russia, from which soldiers (painlessly) died" (quoted from Chroust et al. 1989, p. 61). Other sources, however, cannot confirm such murders (see Sandner 2003, p. 527).

Another, possibly even the most important field of work of the T4 in this intermediate phase was "Aktion Reinhardt". From autumn 1941, the Berlin headquarters supported the construction of the three gas chambers in Poland, Bełżec, Sobibór and Treblinka. Between July 1942 and approximately November 1943, about 1.8 million (primarily Polish) Jews were gassed here (Lehnstaedt 2017). T4 participated with a total of about 100 members (Aly 2013, p. 185; Klee 1986, p. 275f.; Mann 2000, pp. 337, 355f.). Nurses and other employees from Hadamar were also used (Kepplinger 2008, p. 103; Klee 1986, p. 278f.; Lehnstaedt 2017, pp. 34, 41f., 53f.; Sandner 2003, pp. 528ff., 699).

4.2   Characteristics of the Second Murder Phase

Meanwhile, the murders of people with mental and/or psychological illnesses or disabilities continued. A total of more than 100,000 patients were to become victims to the second phase of murder, more than 4400 of them in Hadamar (Faulstich 1998, p. 544; Klee 1986, p. 285; Süß 2007, p. 123). The demonstrative halt to the action thus represented not so much a final cessation. Rather, it was a (short-term) interruption of the killings. However, the killings now took on a new quality: Contrary to what was initially hoped for in the circle of the Central Office, there was no longer a resumption of a centrally controlled or coordinated action (Faulstich 1998, p. 26; Hinz-Wessels et al. 2005, p. 90; Lilienthal 2006b, p. 271f.). Analytically, this second phase therefore testifies to a great ambivalence, complexity and ambiguity of events and results (Süß 2003, p. 311, 2007, p. 123).

Despite this, two central changes compared to the gas murder phase can be emphasized, which are characteristic of the circumstances after the supposed halt: First, regional responsibilities for killing practices increased significantly (Lilienthal 2006a, p. 168, 2010; Süß 2003, p. 351f., 2007; further Aly 2013, p. 180f.). The first initiatives for this change developed in connection with, or as a consequence of, the Sonnenstein meeting held at the end of November 1941 (see Sect. 4.1). At this meeting, the T4 leadership transferred a blanket authorization to kill to a few reliable physicians who were to continue the eugenic operation on a smaller scale in their respective institutions in the future. Whether, where, and how "euthanasia" was carried out thus depended on numerous regional actors – above all the eventual (medical) institution directors, but also the associated supporting authorities as well as state or provincial administrations (Lilienthal 2006a, p. 168f., 2006b, p. 271f.; Sandner 2003, p. 567f., 2006, p. 147). Which institutions ultimately actually participated and to what intensity is thus difficult to determine definitively (Debus et al. 1996, p. 56). In any case, the number of psychiatric institutions involved increased significantly compared to the first phase. In many of the former intermediate institutions, which had almost exclusively served as collection points before, active killing was henceforth carried out (Faulstich 1998, p. 580f.; Lilienthal 2006b, p. 271f.).

On the other hand, the murders in the second phase take on an individualized form (Lilienthal 2006b, p. 271f.). The patients were no longer gassed in larger groups, but starved to death in order to subsequently administer them strong drug overdoses, which in most cases were induced in tablet form and/or as injections. Not infrequently, however, the sick met their deaths as a result of the extreme malnutrition in the psychiatric system (detailed in Faulstich 1998; also Lilienthal 2006a, p. 170; Schmidt-von Blittersdorff et al. 1996, p. 114). In the region of the Nassau District Association, to which Hadamar and its intermediate institutions were subordinate, these hunger and medication killings demonstrably took place as early as 1941 in the Eichberg State Sanatorium and, in all probability, also in Weilmünster (Sandner 2003, p. 569ff.). In Hadamar, on the other hand, the murders did not begin until August 1942, i.e. about a year after the gas killings were originally stopped (Sandner 2006, p. 147). It seems reasonable to assume that the reason why parts of the Hadamar staff were detached to Eichberg and Weilmünster from December 1941 onwards (see Sect. 4.1) was precisely because killing was to resume around that time (Lilienthal 2010, p. 101f.; Sandner 2003, p. 525).

The Central Office's involvement in this second phase of the killings consisted primarily in providing material and, in particular, logistical support for the predominantly regional measures (Hinz-Wessels et al. 2005, p. 90; Kepplinger 2008, p. 106). Whether and to what extent the primary coordination or control of the eugenic projects still lay with the Berlin Central Office in this context is disputed in research (see, for example, Lilienthal 2010; Süß 2007) and, above all, depends on which institutions form the object of investigation. In this context, the LHA Hadamar as a comparatively late-established killing institution in the second phase, has been characterized in historical research as a "special case" (see, for example, Sandner 2003, pp. 607, 649f.). It requires its own, separate considerations that must be raised, with regard to the historical-contextual conditions of the murders of the sick (ibid., p. 569). Here, the questions arise as to when, how and under what circumstances the reopening of the asylum as well as the new transports of the sick occurred (Chap. 5). Secondly, an extension of the empirical puzzle to the murder processes of the second phase inevitably follows: What insights can be gained in the second phase, perhaps in contrast to the usual (mostly historiographical) perspectives, when an organizational sociological interpretation focuses on the murders of the sick (Chap. 6)?

Air War, Disaster Medical Response and the Hadamar Asylum

5

Just as the staff of the Hadamar institution initially continued to be employed (Sect. 4.1), the killing facility also initially remained on "standby". Only when it became increasingly clear in the course of 1942 that the gassing operation could not be continued, were all the alterations originally made by the T4 in Hadamar – including the gas chamber and the crematorium in the basement of the asylum – reversed in early summer. It is striking that these dismantling measures only began when the lease agreement with the Nassau District Association had expired. The agreement was thus not terminated prematurely despite the previous stop because, to all appearances, there was speculation until the very end as to whether the operation could be continued (Lilienthal 2006b, p. 271, 2010, p. 102; Sandner 2003, pp. 608, 610). After the asylum subsequently came into the hands of the District Association, the asylum building was prepared to house 500–600 sick people (Lilienthal 2010, p. 102; see also the testimony of L. Thomas, nursing staff, HHStA/a, p. 60). Functionaries of the Central Office in Berlin, however, promptly contacted repre-

sentatives of the District Association again in order to initiate a reopening of the
Hadamar murder center (Sandner 2003, pp. 609f., 651).[1]

The decision to reintroduce the asylum, the accompanying transports of patients
to be killed later, and the medication killings in Hadamar in general must be seen
in particular against the backdrop of the increasingly intense air raids by the Allies
and the disaster medical response of the Nazi government (Aly 1985b, pp. 31,
56ff.; Faulstich 1998, p. 545; Schmuhl 2011c, p. 231; Süß 2003, p. 353). Because
in threatened or already hit regions the available places in hospitals became increasingly scarce, the responsible regime actors – first and foremost Brandt, who
was closely familiar with the eugenic action – were concerned to create additional
capacities for the benefit of the injured as well as somatically ill. The hospitals,
which in the meantime had been partially disrupted or even destroyed by the bombardments, had to be relieved or replaced at short notice. The regime's disaster
medical care provided for the provision of additional "alternative hospitals" and
medical barracks buildings as the air war progressed, which were generally set up
in or near the psychiatric sanatoriums and nursing homes, most of which were located away from the major cities (Debus et al. 1996, p. 56; Sandner 2003, pp. 631,
648; Schmuhl 2011c, p. 231; Süß 2003, p. 327).

In order to actually be able to guarantee sufficient spatial capacities on the
ground, there were subsequently extensive evacuations of the previous psychiatric
patients in the areas in question (Aly 2013, pp. 177ff., 242f.; Faulstich 1998,

---

[1] Of particular importance for this – and thus for the entire second phase of murder in Hadamar, but also in Eichberg, Herborn and Weilmünster – was the head of the state hospitals (or
rather the asylum department in general) of Hessen-Nassau, Fritz Bernotat, a strong sup-
porter of euthanasia (Chroust et al. 1989, p. 20; Faulstich 1998, p. 541.; Sandner 2003,
pp. 608 f., 625, 2006, p. 140ff.; Winter 1991, p. 91). T4 managing director Dietrich Allers,
the Reich Commissioner for the state hospitals and nursing homes Herbert Linden, as well
as Hans-Joachim Becker, nicknamed "Million-Becker", who, together with the Central Accounting Office, settled accounts for nursing costs with the respective institutions or their
cost bearers, were in contact with Bernotat for the first time (and regularly thereafter) from
around May 1942 in order to reinstall Hadamar as a murder institution and to discuss possible organisational measures with regard to the future murders of the sick (Sandner 2003,
pp. 608f., 641, 2006, p. 148; also Aly 1985a, p. 26ff.).

p. 305; Sandner 2003, p. 587f.).[2] The more severe the consequences of the air war became, the more scarce the available free institutional places became – because time and again not only the injured and physically ill affected by the attacks had to be transferred, but in addition, the psychiatric patients had also to be relocated. In this respect, the Berlin Central Office therefore had a renewed interest in transferring patients to the LHA Hadamar (Lilienthal 2010, p. 103).

From the end of 1942 or the beginning of 1943 at the latest, however, it is no longer possible to speak in this context of planned procedures, but rather, in view of the increasing bombardments, of the Nazi government reacting as quickly as possible to the attacks (Sandner 2003, pp. 611, 632). From this point on, in similar fashion, the transfers of psychiatric patients no longer followed the original selection criteria that had still been applied during the gas murder phase; instead, the deportations depended solely on the air raids and proceeded according to "local need" (Aly 1985b, pp. 31, 56f., 2013, p. 244f.; Faulstich 1998, p. 609; Sandner 2003, p. 631 ff.).[3] In this context, the Reich Commissioner for state hospitals and nursing homes, Herbert Linden (see Sect. 4.1), in particular, decided how many psychiatric patients were to be transferred away, while at the same time the institutions to be evacuated made a selection as to which patients were to join the transports. Typically, some patients, provided they could prove themselves as productive workers, were kept on site (Aly 2013, pp. 21, 179f.; Klee 1986, p. 284; Sandner

---

[2] The deportations and murders of the sick as a result of the regime's emergency management are often referred to in the literature as "Aktion Brandt" (especially in Aly 1985b, p. 56 ff.; for a summarizing account, see Süß 2003, p. 311f.). This description derives from the fact that Karl Brandt, who was appointed as „Generalkommissar für das Sanitäts- und Gesundheitswesen"(General Commissioner for Medical and Health Services) at the time, was responsible for the creation of said additional medical capacities, specifically the barracks buildings. In research, however, this term is disputed (Sandner 2003, pp. 587., 704f.; Süß 2003, p. 315ff., 2007, p. 123). Its use becomes problematic not least because the precise notion of a "Aktion Brandt" varies from author to author, leading to differences in usage and understanding (see, for example, Faulstich 1998, pp. 305ff., 609ff.; a brief overview in Sandner 2003, p. 587f.). I therefore refrain from using this misleading term in the further course of the work.

[3] Although the T4 registration forms were continued after the stop and in some cases even intensified by formal requests from the Central Office, they never regained the relevance they once had and were intended to have (Faulstich 1998, pp. 296f., 310; Hinz-Wessels et al. 2005, p. 89f.; Lilienthal 2010, p. 102). In principle, it cannot be assumed that the registration forms – perhaps far from some of the early transports between July and November 1942 – still served to select the later victims (Sandner 2003, p. 634f.; but see for a – now probably outdated – counter perspective Debus et al. 1996; Schmidt-von-Blittersdorff et al. 1996). Finally, the obligation to complete the registration forms was finally abolished in August 1944, presumably for war-related reasons (Debus et al. 1996, p. 51; Sandner 2003, p. 630f.).

2003, pp. 506f., 633f.; see also Süß 2007, pp. 126, 128). The resulting transfers (and later killings) were thus only subject to eugenic calculations to a limited extent. Instead, they were carried out primarily in regards to work ability or productivity (Aly 1985b, p. 56f., 2013, p. 245; Faulstich 1998, pp. 545, 609, 625f.).

It was possible to determine which institutional rooms were still available for the psychiatric patients thanks to previous organizational and bureaucratic measures (for this see, for example, Aly 2013, p. 243; Faulstich 1998, p. 309; Sandner 2003, p. 635f.), which began immediately after Linden took office (Chroust et al. 1989, p. 66; Hirschinger 2001, p. 147; Sandner 2003, p. 516f.). From then on, the regional institutions in particular played an important role because Linden, despite his high official position, could not freely dispose of their capacities (see also Süß 2003, p. 316). The Reich Commissioner for state hospitals and nursing homes (or rather the Central Office in general) was thus dependent on the willingness of the institutions to cooperate. The Nassau District Association in particular proved to be a very cooperative and willing partner (Faulstich 1998, p. 308f.; Lilienthal 2010, p. 104; Sandner 2003, p. 637ff.; see also Sect. 6.1.5), which is why T4 director Allers later thanked Bernotat in writing for his "obligingness in accepting the mentally ill" (quoted in Sandner 2003, p. 620). No further analysis is required to be clear about what was meant by such an "acceptance" (ibid.).

As a result of the mutual agreements between the Nassau District Association (above all Bernotat) and the T4 headquarters in Berlin (in particular Linden, Becker, Brandt and Allers), close cooperation developed between the parties on the premise of completing the procedures as quickly and broadly as possible (Lilienthal 2010, p. 103). As soon as agreement could be reached in an individual case on the acceptance of a (further) transport, the "Charitable Foundation for the Transport of Patients, Inc." (*Gemeinnützige Kranken-Transport GmbH*) – in short: "Gekrat" –, a (bogus) company created by T4 in the first murder phase and used in many cases before, took over all patient transports for transfers from institutions located outside the Nassau District Association (Aly 2013, p. 179f.; Lilienthal 2010, p. 105f.; Sandner 2003, pp. 640, 652f.; Schmidt-von Blittersdorff et al. 1996, pp. 101, 104f.).

During its active period, a total of 63 larger transports (i.e. comprising more than 20 persons) can be identified for the Hadamar LHA between 1942 and 1945 (Schmidt-von Blittersdorff et al. 1996, p. 103f.). These can be divided into three central categories (for the following explanations, see Lilienthal 2010, p. 103ff.; also Schmidt-von Blittersdorff et al. 1996, p. 103f.): First, there were several transports between November 1942 and April 1943 in which over 600 patients from the intermediate institutions were transferred to Hadamar and murdered. Originally, these people were to be liquidated as part of the gassing phase, but it did not happen in terms of time because of the halt. These people now arrived at their originally intended destination with a delay of about one to one and a half years (on this, see also Faulstich 1998, p. 549; Schmidt-von Blittersdorff et al. 1996, p. 101f.). The transport to Hadamar was arranged by Gekrat, while the Central Accounting Office for State Hospitals and Nursing Homes (*Zentralverrechnungsstelle*) settled the nursing costs. Secondly, there were numerous transports between June 1943 and June 1944 that were directly related to the air war measures described above. Three deportations in August 1942 from Bremen and the Rhineland preceded this period (Faulstich 1998, p. 619; Werner 1991, p. 141). Many patients of this second category were accommodated in one of the other institutions of the District Association (Eichberg, Weilmünster or Scheuern). Here, too, the Gekrat as well as the Central Accounting Office were involved accordingly.

A last type of transports took place between September 1943 and March 1945, i.e. until the euthanasia was finally ended by the invasion of American troops in Hadamar. These were exclusively intra-district transfers, in which the sick were transported from the nearby institutions of the District Association to Hadamar. In this respect, the involvement of Gekrat and the Central Accounting Office can only be ascertained up to the point of arrival at the district-owned institutions, but not for the onward intra-district transfers (Sandner 2003, p. 644f.). In a sense, this was a return to the system of intermediate institutions from the first phase, which allowed the parties involved to place a large number of psychiatric patients in the institutions of the District Association (Faulstich 1998, p. 554ff.). In comparison to the gas murders, however, a central difference lay in the fact that in the meantime murder was also actively carried out in the intermediate institutions (Sect. 4.2), i.e. these "more modern intermediate institutions" sometimes themselves functioned as "final stations" for many of the patients (Faulstich 1998, p. 554; Sandner 2003, pp. 645, 702). However, they retained their original form as a collection point or intermediate station because the mortality rates in Hadamar were significantly higher than in Eichberg, Weilmünster and above all Scheuern, for which it has not yet been possible to prove involvement in the medication murders (Sandner 2003, p. 644f.). In the event of high occupancy rates in the intermediate institutions, patients were accordingly transferred to the Hadamar LHA (ibid.).[4]

---

[4]The mortality rates in Hadamar were 59.9% (502 of 838 patients) for the year 1942, 75.2% (1583 of 2105 patients) for 1943, 75.8% (1903 of 2511 patients) for 1944 as well as 52.2% for 1945 (430 of 823 patients). Despite the lower mortality rate compared to the previous years, the value from 1945 is particularly astonishing, because the murders had already been (finally) stopped in April due to the war ending (Faulstich 1998, p. 544, 616). In percentage terms, the LHA Hadamar is the institution in which by far the most people succumbed to drug-related murder (ibid., p. 583f.).

Between 13 and 18 August 1942, the first patients arrived in Hadamar after the reopening of the asylum (Aly 2013, p. 244f.; Schmidt-von Blittersdorff et al. 1996, p. 103; Süß 2007, p. 125). At this point, all details had been settled between the Berlin officials and the Nassau District Association, for example with regard to staffing, the billing of care costs, and the provision of various equipment (Sandner 2003, p. 610f., 2006, p. 148).[5] The (extremely important) task of the Central Office was primarily the regular mass transfer of sick persons from all over the German Reich to the LHA Hadamar (Faulstich 1998, p. 545; Sandner 2003, p. 626f.). However, the tasks on site, such as the selection of victims or the planning and execution of the final killing procedures, were the responsibility of the staff of the institution itself (Lilienthal 2010, p. 109f.; see Chap. 6).

Therefore – and in contrast to, for example, Friedlander (1997, p. 253) –, the LHA Hadamar cannot be analysed in isolation from the central structures that operated in Berlin.[6] It also seems inappropriate to speak in this context of a "wild euthanasia" – a term often postulated in research (for example, Benedict and Kuhla 1999; Winter 1991; also Hirschinger 2001, p. 152, FN 287), which illustrate the murders of the sick after the halt of the action as entirely unregulated and uncoordinated

[5]Although the murder of the sick was certainly accepted in many cases (and especially as time went on), it can be assumed that some of the original asylums were not informed, or at best only conditionally informed, about what would happen during a transport to Hadamar (Sandner 2003, p. 574; Süß 2003, p. 332, 2007, p. 127f.). This can be said with a fair degree of certainty, for example, for the first transports from the Rhineland in August 1942: in view of the various rumours, the then head of the Rhineland institution, Walter Creutz, visited the LHA Hadamar himself before any of his patients were transferred, in order to check whether any of the sick would be killed. To all appearances, the asylum seemed to have reached a psychiatric ordinariness by then (Süß 2003, p. 332; Werner 1991, p. 141; also Chroust et al. 1989, p. 70; Sandner 2003, p. 611f.). In fact, however, a large number of these patients were dead only a few weeks later (Süß 2007, p. 125). When a total of 43 of the transferred patients were already reported as deceased in September, Creutz inquired about the strikingly high mortality rate in Hadamar. The reply of the doctor in charge in Hadamar, Adolf Wahlmann (more in Chap. 6), stated in this regard, among other things: "I cannot, however, reconcile it with my National Socialist attitude to apply any medical measures, be they medicinal or of any other kind, so that the lives of these individuals, who are complete failures for human society, are prolonged" (quoted from Schmidt-von Blittersdorff et al. 1996, p. 112). Süß's remarks (2007, p. 127f.) suggest at one point that Creutz would have inquired in advance about the chances of survival of the sick, but this is not correct (see, for example, Schmidt-von Blittersdorff et al. 1996, p. 111f.; Werner 1991, p. 141). Also contrary to the description by Süß (2003, p. 332, 2007, p. 128), it was not the institutional director who wrote this answer. Wahlmann was regarded in the Hadamar hierarchy as chief physician, subordinate to the actual head of the institution, state inspector Alfons Klein (Faulstich 1998, p. 615; Kintner 1948, p. 16f.; Sandner 2003, p. 612ff.).

[6]To be precise, Friedlander says the murders in asylums such as "Eichberg, Hadamar, Kalmenhof, Meseritz-Obrawalde and Tiegenhof [...] were in fact decentralized and chaotic" (1997, p. 253).

measures (Süß 2003, p. 311).[7] Much more plausible is the portrayal of Hadamar as a *supra-regional killing center,* which acted in close cooperation with the Central Office and thus advanced to an (unofficial) successor to the aborted, centrally controlled and coordinated operation of the gas murder phase (Faulstich 1998, pp. 544, 580f.; Lilienthal 2006a, p. 16, 2010, p. 110; Sandner 2003, p. 608, 2006, p. 147f.; also Süß 2003, p. 327). That the LHA Hadamar was based on such a calculation from the beginning in the second murder phase cannot be asserted with absolute certainty (Süß 2003, p. 353), but is at least suggested by the composition of the Reich-wide and chronologically coordinated transports (Schmidt-von Blittersdorff et al. 1996, pp. 103f.; also Lilienthal 2010), is further shown by the close cooperation with the Central Office or its affiliated institutions (Gekrat as well as the Central Accounting Office), and is additionally evident from the fact that only a few days after the reopening, the first patients from Bremen and the Rhineland were already admitted through Gekrat (Sandner 2003, p. 610.). This interpretation is further supported by the fact that besides the first three transports immediately after Hadamar's reopening – which arrived as a result of the air raids – it were precisely those patients who were able to temporarily escape the intended or planned death by gas due to the halt of the operation who were transferred and killed. Last but not least, the enormously high (and comparatively also by far the highest) mortality rate (for this, see FN 4 in this chapter) also points to a procedure that was carried out in a planned manner from the very beginning (Faulstich 1998, p. 544).

It could be objected that within the framework of the third transport batches, internal district transfers were carried out, i.e. the associated killings served solely or primarily to reduce regional overcrowding with the simultaneous knowledge of the T4 Central Office (for this perspective, see Süß 2007; also Süß 2003, p. 352f.). However, it must be taken into account that, on the one hand, these internal deportations were also preceded by some out-of-district (pre-)transfers from other facilities (see above), for whose cost accounting the Central Accounting Office was responsible yet again (Lilienthal 2010, p. 107). On the other hand, this last transport category (September 1943 to March 1945) is to be interpreted additionally or especially in the context of an increasingly worsening war situation, because longer transports through the then German Reich were probably no longer possible, if only in view of the destroyed transport routes (ibid., pp. 108, 110). In any case, some regional or intra-district transfers are not per se incompatible with a more centralistic view of the murders in Hadamar during the second phase (further implications in Sect. 7.1).

---

[7] For further perspectives, see Sandner (2003, p. 628). In his study of the Altscherbitz institution, Hirschinger (2001, p. 151f.) was unable to conclusively clarify whether the drug murders carried out after 1941 were centrally or regionally controlled measures.

The Second Murder Phase in Hadamar

In addition to the changes at the organizational level of the murders of the sick, there was also a transformation in the method of killing at the Hadamar LHA. The transformation from the comparatively anonymous gas killings to a now significantly more direct and personal form of euthanasia through the deliberate overdose of medication was inevitably accompanied by some additional inhibitions, following the explanations about the fundamental avoidance of confrontational situations in the first phase (Sect. 3.2.5):

> I realized that I should now kill immediately ... It took a long time until I had made up my mind to give the tablets to the certain sick people. (statement Zachow, nursing staff, quoted after Wettlaufer 1996, p. 300)

> I have to add though, that for the most part, most of the personnel did not agree with the action. I even saw a head nurse (meaning Irmgard Huber, DF) who had tears in her eyes. She stood there when the first cars arrived and cried bitterly. One saw it in the faces but no one dared say anything. (statement by Losen, technical staff, quoted from Benedict 2003, p. 68)

In fact, however, neither the changes described above nor other associated obstacles – which were certainly felt to different degrees depending on the individual – were able to stop the killings. On the contrary, the killing in the asylum continued in a modified manner. It was not limited to individual exceptional cases on the part of the perpetrator or victim, but was (still or once again) the entire purpose of the Hadamar murder centre.

How such consistency could be maintained, however, requires explanation. On the basis of the previous findings, it seems reasonable to assume that the practices in the context of the drug murders were also characterized by a certain, not immediately recognizable structure or regularity, which must be analytically elaborated and examined more closely. Based on the chosen approach of the present study, it is therefore primarily of interest in the following whether more general patterns can be observed or reconstructed that formed the basis of the killings in the second phase following the gas murders.

For this purpose, after a descriptive presentation of the basic course of the drug murders (Sect. 6.1), I will elaborate some characteristics of the killing process within the institution that are worth emphasizing and that were significant for the conditions and interpretations of the staff (Sects. 6.1.1–6.1.6).[1] A combination of these aspects will make clear that a certain, constantly repeated killing pattern can also be observed in the medication killings, which was valid in this form at least for the murder of *German* psychiatric patients until the invasion of the American troops in Hadamar in March 1945. The theoretically and empirically validated assumption derived from this is that an explanation of the medication murders is based on the staff's *remembered knowledge structures* or *interpretations* as well as the *continuation of previous interactional experiences* (Sect. 6.2). Whether and to what extent this thesis is also plausible beyond the German patients or even the reference case of Hadamar will be discussed later (Sect. 7.1).

6.1 The Medication Murders in Hadamar: The Basic Sequence of Events

With the transports arriving from August 1942 onwards, the eugenic action in Hadamar was continued after an interruption of about 1 year. In contrast to the events of the gas murder phase, however, the patients were no longer killed at once or as quickly as possible. In the second phase, contact between the nursing staff and the patients was no longer limited to a few hours at most or to a short escort to the gas chamber (Wettlaufer 1996, p. 306), so that episodes of nursing normality were established, especially when the patients arrived:

A: I received them just like the other patients, and saw to it that they would get into a good bed. […] The transport had arrived and had to be received. […]

Q: Did you help the people?

---

[1] A more detailed analytical examination of the bureaucratic post-processing of the murders, which is largely similar to the gas murder phase, is omitted – my focus here, apart from the description of the basic and repeating sequence of events (Sect. 6.1), is solely on the immediate killing procedure.

A: Yes, I put them to bed. I could not let them stand outside. (statement Huber, nursing staff, quoted after Kintner 1948, p. 116f.)

Although the main task at the Hadamar LHA continued to be the killing of eligible patients, actual, at least selective, nursing treatment in the true sense of the term can be observed – presumably precisely because of the longer stay (e.g. Wettlaufer 1996, pp. 305, 320f., 327f.; see also Sect. 6.1.1). After their arrival, the people were divided up into different wards. The differentiation criteria on which this was based included gender on the one hand and the respective person's ability to work on the other.

Subsequently, in connection with the murders, a procedure developed which was to be maintained in this (or at least very similar) form until the (final) stop of euthanasia (Chroust et al. 1989, p. 71): At around 9 a.m., daily conferences were held between head physician Dr. Adolf Wahlmann, head nurse Heinrich Ruoff, and head nurse Irmgard Huber (statement Blum, technical staff, Kintner 1948, p. 84; statement J. Thomas, office staff, Kintner 1948, p. 25). The ward nurse L. Thomas was involved as a substitute (statement Dr. Wahlmann, chief physician, HHStA/a, p. 79). In these joint discussions, it was discussed and decided who was to be "euthanized" in a timely manner on the basis of Wahlmann's own rounds, which were conducted on a regular or even daily basis, possibly also on the basis of information provided by the ward nurses,[2] and, above all, taking into account the personnel files and medical histories of the patients (see also the testimony of Dr. Wahlmann, chief physician, HHStA/a, p. 38). The selection was made primarily according to the working capacity of the sick, and if necessary also according to their need for care as well as the associated expenses and costs (Chroust et al. 1989, p. 71f.; Sandner 2003, p. 623). The final (death) verdict was always decided by Dr. Wahlmann himself as the only physician in the institution (Schmidt-von Blittersdorff et al. 1996, p. 114f.; see also statement Huber, nursing staff, Kintner 1948, p. 129):

Whether other sisters made suggestions? I don't know. That the doctor said of his own accord that it was her and her turn? Whether he just said, it's the turn of this one and that one – oh yes, that he called upon the people, that's what I saw during the rounds. (statement by L. Thomas, nursing staff, HHStA/a, p. 61)

---

[2] In view of witness statements to the contrary, it is not entirely clear whether suggestions for the intended measures were also made in part by the ward nurses and what influence these suggestions, if they actually existed, may have had (see, for example, Benedict 2003, p. 69f.; Schmidt-von Blittersdorff et al. 1996, p. 114; Winter 1991, p. 102).

> The nurses, like Gneiser, etc., they wrote down the bad cases on a piece of paper, and she presented it to me, and the doctor said I should present the medical history, and I had the personnel files given to me, presented them, and after that the doctor decided. […] That went through every day. He would sometimes say such and such was so lapsed. Usually it went in the form that the ward nurses issued the slips, the slips were presented to me and I passed them on to Dr. Wahlmann. What the doctor decided, I gave back. Verbal or written decision from the doctor? Who was to be killed? He told me that and I was supposed to write them down. (statement Huber, nursing staff, HHStA/a, p. 49)

In the context of this conference, Wahlmann thus informed both head nurses about his decisions made on (allegedly) medical grounds and passed on the corresponding information. The tasks of the head nurses now consisted of taking down the names in writing and passing the slips of paper on to the corresponding ward manager in whose care the victim was (Benedict 2003, p. 69f.; Chroust et al. 1989, p. 71f.; Schmidt-von Blittersdorff et al. 1996, p. 114f.). It can be assumed that the exact dosage of medication depended on the respective condition of the patients and was thus often left to the executing ward nurses (Schmidt-von Blittersdorff et al. 1996, p. 114f.). Chief physician Wahlmann described this procedure as follows:

> I went through the ward every morning. The conference, it was 9 o'clock in the morning, the head nurses or a deputy were there. I held the conference. We discussed the general at first and every few days, maybe once a week, the cases were picked out based on their medical files. […] We discussed beforehand who could be taken on like that today, in the conference at 9 o'clock. […] The conference was before the rounds. It may be that I said: this one and that one will be done tomorrow, and that these cases were then discussed the other morning at the conference. I think one of the head nurses gave me a slip of paper for those that were to be done today, following on from yesterday's conference. Whether the head nurse also gave names independently? I don't think she needed to. I talked to almost every sick person every day. It was a good thing to do. I'd go through at lunchtime and look at people. You must imagine a pretty intimate life there with the sick. I knew what was going on, and in this way a lot of things came about by themselves; the head nurses helped out. Now we discussed the case and then I decided whose turn it should be, and I had the female head nurse write it down on a piece of paper. She took this note with her and gave it to her staff. I myself had nothing to do with the staff, I had no authority whatsoever, I had no say in the matter. The whole order, also the euthanasia itself, happened without my intervention. I merely wrote down the medication. (statement by Wahlmann, chief physician, HHStA/a, p. 26f.)

The killing order associated with the passed-on notes was ultimately carried out by the nurses and orderlies working in the wards where the victims were located

(Sandner 2003, p. 623). In this context, the patients to be executed were apparently (at least partially) transferred to a so-called "death" or "slumber room" (Schmidt-von Blittersdorff et al. 1996, pp. 108, 113; Winter 1991, p. 102; also Friedlander 1997, p. 264).

The actual method of murder involved the distribution of overdosed tablets, usually in the afternoon or evening, if necessary immediately before bedtime, by the staff who had to perform night duty that night (Winter 1991, p. 102). In many cases, this dosage was sufficient to cause death in patients who were already mostly weakened and malnourished. However, if the patients were still alive the next morning, the nurses on early duty administered a definitely lethal injection (Chroust et al. 1989, p. 71f.; Schmidt-von Blittersdorff et al. 1996, p. 114f.; Winter 1991, p. 102; see also Zachow's statement, nursing staff, Kintner 1948, p. 20):

> [...] Then the dying started. The note came at night and the medicines were on the table. The patients were very frightened. In the morning the ward nurse Willich came, sees 2 patients still asleep. He asked me what was wrong with them. I said, well, I had sent them to the lavatory. He prepared the syringes and gave them the shot. He said it was better than waking them up. I experienced this again when he came with Klein. (statement by Lückoff, nursing staff, HHStA/a, p. 88)

> Killings? It has already happened during my on-call duty that there was a note on the table, some liquid in the bottle, and it said that the patient – gets another glass of the solution. I then also gave that. (statement by Reuter, nursing staff, HHStA/a, p. 68)

In the second phase, too, a bureaucratic processing of the events, provided with false information, began after the murders. Telegrams were sent to the relatives stating that the patient concerned was dying or had succumbed to corresponding (again fictitious) circumstances (Schmidt-von Blittersdorff et al. 1996, p. 114f.). Those who reacted quickly enough to the short-notice notifications had the chance to participate in an individual burial and to have the bodies of his or her relatives transferred to the home town or for cremation. The usual practice, however, was to entomb the lightly or unclothed bodies of victims in mass graves without burial. With this new method of burial, those involved reacted to the smoking chimney and the difficulties of the first phase resulting from the cremation of corpses (Friedlander 1997, p. 264; Lilienthal 2006a, p. 169f.; Sandner 2003, p. 623f.; Schmidt-von Blittersdorff et al. 1996, p. 114f.; see also Chap. 4).

6.1.1   Medical Primacy

With regard to the killing procedure described, it is first of all striking that the method selected was oriented towards being as "medical a method of liquidation" as possible (Welzer 2005, pp. 127, 129): Patients were not killed by the use of excessive physical force or weapons, for example, but by administering – to make use here of the common euphemism used by nurses – "medicine" to those who were bedridden and/or physically weak or ill. Thus, recourse was made to a course of action that seemed justifiable to the staff in view of their professional background and the ethos associated with it (ibid., p. 38), namely "healing by extermination":

> After all, I know from my own experience that an injection, when you are ill, is a pleasant thing. (statement by Kneissler, nursing staff, quoted from Wettlaufer 1996, p. 320)

> During my work in the sanatorium and nursing home I had also become acquainted with the serious cases and had also seen quite a number of terminal patients, including patients who ate their own excrement. I therefore had understanding for wanting to put such sick people out of their misery. I had seen that life was nothing but torture for them. (statement by Korsch, nursing staff, Wettlaufer 1996, p. 309)

In general, the entire procedure, beginning with the selection of the sick and ending with the conspicuously clinically pure nature of the murders (Sandner 2003, p. 623), is based on an apparent medical primacy. In view of the fact that it was primarily the institutions internal chief physician who, after allegedly appropriate considerations of the medical records and medical visits were made, had to decide which patients were ultimately to be murdered, genuine intentions were at least suggested (ibid., p. 616; see also Kneissler's statement, nursing staff, Wettlaufer 1996, p. 320). Accordingly, the nurses Huber and Zachow described, for example, that the patients to be murdered were always chosen conscientiously and according to factual considerations – or, put different: via medical necessities (Wettlaufer 1996, pp. 307f., 326).

In this context, the head physician Wahlmann in particular was attested to warm-hearted treatment of the sick, which earned him the nickname "Jesus Christ" (Sandner 2003, p. 613f.). Evidence suggests that a demeanor oriented toward such norms was also expected on part of the staff. To a certain extent, this (supposed) medical attitude was expressed in the already mentioned, in relation to the killing order actually paradoxical conception of the nursing staff, according to which they were "obliged to the closest consideration of the medical prescription for the most careful care of the sick" (statement Kneissler, nursing staff, quoted after Wettlaufer 1996, p. 320): "The care of the sick lying in the last stage required the greatest sacrifice. The sick were thoroughly cared for, as I always used to do" (statement Zachow, nursing staff, ibid., p. 306). Meanwhile, the nurse Richtstein was released from her duties after a short time, because one had to "comply with the wishes of the sick" (statement Huber, nursing staff, HHStA/a, p. 74) and Richtstein would not have been able to do so.

The fact that, at least in individual cases, genuine nursing and care tasks were performed is by no means to be interpreted solely as a form of conscience relief (Wettlaufer 1996, p. 306). Instead, we find here an indication that a certain moral (pseudo) integrity determined the regulated procedures, so that in the subjective view of the perpetrators the practices could be understood less as murder (Welzer 2005, pp. 38, 46, 262) than as legitimate and medically legitimized euthanasia. The significance of this aspect in the context of the everyday killing work of the nursing staff is expressed precisely in those places where individual nurses deviated from the standardised procedure and, for example, became violent towards the sick. This additional use of violence was met with great incomprehension among the staff (Wettlaufer 1996, p. 305). Especially the orderlies Ruoff and Willig stood out negatively with regard to possible abuse or even rape of some female patients: "Especially the head orderly Willig was very robust. He would have liked to take us nurses to the concentration camp as well" (statement by Gumbmann, nursing staff, quoted from Wettlaufer 1996, p. 305).

I refer so explicitly to this additional use of violence, which is perceived as problematic, because this initially seems contradictory in view of the existing organizational purpose – which was the destruction of human life. However, the fact that the fisticuffs of some nurses were portrayed in such a negative light is, in my opinion, due to the fact that this form of violence was not included in the legal and organisational framework that legitimised it from the perspective of the actors, i.e. these actions took place far away from the killing programme and were therefore much more likely to be attributable to the respective nurses as *personal* misconduct (see also Sect. 3.2.3). The ethos of healing and redemption projected onto the tasks could no longer be upheld in these cases – which staged the use of physical violence as particularly bad in comparison to their own organisationally protected approach and thus led to the relativisation of their own actions. This is reflected again in the following testimony, when a nurse appears concerned about the strangulation of a sick person, but not about the lethal injection administered to the patient beforehand:

Q: You stated a sick person was strangled?

A: One evening Sister Irmgard came to me and was very upset. She told me that a patient had received an injection but had not yet died from it by the time the doctors arrived for rounds. Nurse Willich, she said, had not even given the patient time to die and had held his throat closed. Sister Irmgard was horrified and indignant at this, and declared that it was appalling to her to live among such people. […]

Q: Did she refuse?

A: She was horrified by what had happened. She was a religious person and from this point of view she went through a severe inner conflict. (statement T. Vogel, witness, HHStA/a, p. 242)

6.1.2   The Hierarchization of Patients

The (alleged) medical primacy underlying the murders also emerged as a result of an apparently careful selection of the sick, on the basis of which mercy killing was to be granted only to those who were affected by the selection criteria provided for this purpose (Wettlaufer 1996, p. 326; see also Sect. 6.1.4). In this context, for example, one nurse expressed the view "that the National Socialists were serious about their social programme and that they could and would also help in great hardships […]" (statement by Margot R.-G., nursing staff, quoted after Wettlaufer 1996, p. 309). The often accompanying indifferent or even approving reactions of relatives of the sick did the rest to strengthen the nursing staff in this way of thinking (see, for example, the statements of the sisters Margot R.-G., Kneissler and Huber, nursing staff, Wettlaufer 1996, pp. 309, 321, 326).

An initial selection of patients, at least from the perspective of the staff, apparently also took place in the second murder phase even before the patients were brought to the institution (Schmidt-von Blittersdorff et al. 1996, p. 113):

Correspondence with Berlin? Yes, we had taken care of that. Above all, when transports came, they were reported immediately to Berlin; I did that on behalf of Klein. A list went to Tiergartenstraße 4 and a list to the Central Accounting Office, which was also in Berlin […]. Everything that was transferred to Hadamar, name, date of birth, the institution where they came from. […] Authorizations from Berlin? I only know that the transports were still checked by the Foundation. […] I can only remember larger transports, from Warstein, from Klosterhofen, from Eichberg. […] Whether the transports from Berlin were checked? I know that the transports were reported to Berlin; that is my assumption that they were checked there. (statement J. Thomas, office staff, HHStA/a, p. 129)

Although such a presumed (pre-)selection, as described (Chap. 5), was in fact no longer carried out by the Berlin authorities, the notion of an initial selection was nevertheless certainly not entirely wrong, since the institutions that were evacuated in the course of the air raids kept patients fit for work on their premises, while it was precisely those who were considered unfit for work or who required comparatively greater care who had to join a transport (Sandner 2003, p. 692; Schmidt-von Blittersdorff et al. 1996, p. 113). This idea gets even more validation due to the fact that the original displacement and transfer of psychiatric patients in favour of the somatically ill and injured was nothing other than the result of yet another inferior treatment of the stigmatised as well as incapacitated patients (Süß 2003, p. 327).

Moreover, mainly for war-related reasons, the already financially strapped psychiatric establishment in Germany was affected by even more drastic cuts in the available budgetary resources and, above all, food rations, so that psychiatric patients in many cases either succumbed to starvation – sometimes even in the course of the transports to Hadamar – without deliberate intent, or arrived at the asylum in a physically enormously poor, infectious, almost exclusively bedridden condition (Faulstich 1998, p. 548; Schmidt-von Blittersdorff et al. 1996, p. 111; see also the statement of Wahlmann, chief physician, HHStA/a, p. 28; similarly already in Sect. 3.1). In this sense, from the staff's point of view, mercy killing could be understood to a certain extent:

> Whether I thought if it was right to stop feeding the mentally ill in that state? Yes, I have already thought about that. But the patients we had were so badly off physically that sometimes they could no longer stand at all, and most of them starved to death. And in my opinion it was a blessing that such people died as quickly as possible. (statement by Reuter, nursing staff, HHStA/a, p. 69)

Of particular importance in this context, however, was the further-reaching hierarchization of the sick *within* the institution according to "healthy" (i.e. primarily capable of work) and "mentally ill" (i.e. incapable of work) patients, so that the former could be "spared the measures ordered by Berlin" (statement by Huber, nursing staff, quoted from Wettlaufer 1996, p. 325; also Benedict 2003, p. 69):

> At first it was a real mess, we had no real overview of the patients. The beds were occupied so that everyone had a bed, and Herr Obermedizinalrat began to sort out what was unclean, so that they were sent to other wards. We had so many bed-wetters that one could not even step into the hall in the morning, puddles were lying around, excrement was thrown around. (statement by L. Thomas, nursing staff, HHStA/a, p. 60)

Q: Which sick people did she give sleeping pills to? Which ones were seriously ill or feeble-minded. What kind of sick people were they?

A: Mentally they were on a very low level. They sat there all day and didn't do a handshake. We had to dress them. [...] If they were quiet patients, they were not used to the tablets. (statement by Zielke, nursing staff, HHStA/a, p. 101)

In my opinion, the patients thus eliminated were all seriously ill and no longer quite fit to live; all the others had been separated out and transferred to the work wards. (statement by Huber, nursing staff, quoted from Wettlaufer 1996, p. 326)

In view of this selection, both external and internal to the institution, it is therefore difficult to speak of arbitrary killings, contrary to what is usually presented in numerous other studies (e.g. George 2006, p. 236; Lilienthal 2006a, p. 171, 2006b, p. 271f.; some remarks were also made in Chap. 5). Admittedly, in view of the air-war-related necessities, the transports of patients controlled from Berlin were carried out much more arbitrarily than in the first phase, but the internal institution procedures described above testify to the opposite: the daily rounds and conferences, which directly served to separate those incapable of work, those in need of care, and "life unworthy of life" from the "serviceable," operated on the basis of selection criteria that had already been of great importance in the gas murder phase. In this respect, one can observe in Hadamar a (primarily war-related) radicalized or intensified, but not an arbitrary selection and killing, therefore rather an imitation of previously valid as well as legitimized criteria on the basis of an unambiguous *hierarchization* of patients (Süß 2003, p. 327). This can be seen, among other things, in the fact that people demonstrably survived or were able to survive if and as long as they were able to work (Daum 1996, p. 197): "No persons able to work were killed" (statement Zielke, nursing staff, HHStA/a, p. 98). In fact, those who were able to pursue occupations in the institution or were capable of "temporary work" – patients capable of work were loaned out to shops or the like for a fee payable to the institution or the District Association – were not only not killed, but kept alive (longer) by better rations at the expense of the patients incapable of work (Daum 1996, pp. 195f., 205; Faulstich 1998, p. 546; Schmidt-von Blittersdorff et al. 1996, p. 105ff.).

Similar to the first phase, the motto was: as long as a person could still provide productive services for the institution's economy, that person's life was spared at least for the time being. Such a categorization of patients, based on an apparent medical precedent, inevitably conformed the staff to the "socio-historical, cultural and situational settings" (Welzer 2005, p. 87) in which they found themselves, so that previously existing ideas of the staff about "life worth living" as well as "life unworth living" still seemed plausible. The selection of patients, however, was not randomly made, but was based on a corresponding cost-benefit calculation instead.

6.1.3   Personnel Continuities

The fact that there was a fundamental familiarity with the (modified) tasks can be seen not only in the continuation and confirmation of old ideas about psychiatric patients (Sects. 6.1.1 and 6.1.2), but also in the fact that almost exclusively former personnel was either retained or newly recruited employees could draw on old experience in the murder of the sick (Süß 2003, p. 353). Within a short period of time, in August 1942, the District Association jointly reorganized the personnel conditions in the LHA Hadamar in (yet another) close cooperation with the Berlin Central Office (Sandner 2003, p. 618ff.). From then on, employees of the District Association worked in the killing centre to the greatest possible extent, while the Central Office helped out with any nurses as well as with other (service-obligated) administrative employees (ibid., pp. 612, 616f.). Although staffing levels were often tight and this problem was increasingly intensified in view of the advancing war and the associated military conscription of male personnel (ibid., p. 617; also Sect. 6.1.6), those responsible evidently continued to attach great importance to recruiting or retaining politically loyal, appropriately trained personnel with a positive attitude towards the eugenic campaign (ibid., p. 617). This can be stated especially for the hierarchically higher positions – for example the ward sisters (Huber, Gumbmann and L. Thomas) or the head nurse (also Huber) (ibid., p. 618f.).[3] Meanwhile, the head nurse's request for dismissal was rejected by the institution management because "no *new* staff could be needed in the institution" (statement by Huber, nursing staff, HHStA/a, p. 51, emphasis DF).

Many of the previous staff members whom the District Association had seconded to T4 and who had tried their hand at euthanasia during the first murder phase were now re-contracted in the subsequent period. In addition, there were some people – among others the head nurse Ruoff as well as ward nurse Heinrich W., who were also members of the SA – who had not previously been seconded to T4, but who remained in the Hadamar asylum and were employed elsewhere (Sandner 2003, p. 616). Therefore, it seems reasonable to assume that already socialized staff members were deliberately used to engage in further or – especially in comparison to the first murder phase – more serious illegal practices. After all, they have proven that they were capable of the demanded requests (Kühl 2020a, p. 114f.; see also Sect. 3.3 on the intensification of expectations). In view of the

---

[3] Incidentally, this familiarity also applied to the chief physician Wahlmann (newly hired for the second phase), who had worked in the asylums of the Nassau District Association for several decades and had accordingly also always been familiar with the eugenic campaign and demonstrably convinced of its correctness (Sandner 2003, p. 613ff.).

continuities in personnel and the numerous experiences that the Hadamar cadre had already gained in the first murders of the sick, it can be concluded that the medically legitimized killing process was not able to develop an alien or overly threatening character even despite the switch to a much more direct method (Welzer 2005, pp. 124, 169), but that it was a rather normalized expectation of action – albeit certainly difficult or maybe even more difficult to exercise.[4]

6.1.4   Responsibility Diffusion

For all the discussion about the question of how central the euthanasia measures still were (or were not) after the second murder phase, it must be kept in mind that the Hadamar institution was still an organization in the sense defined above (Chap. 2), i.e. with corresponding formal hierarchies and behavioral expectations. Accordingly, the usual, strict chains of command and hierarchy in the asylum can also be observed in the second murder phase: Bernotat and Klein, for example, but also the deputy head of the T4 personnel department, Arnold Oels, visited the asylum early after Hadamar's reopening in August 1942 in order to convey a clear killing order to the employees on site (Sandner 2003, p. 622; Wettlaufer 1996, p. 299).

Particularly instructive for the behaviour of the nursing staff were again the instructions of the asylum doctor. In view of the basically identical (or at least very similar) professional ethos as well as the medical primacy underlying the killings (Sect. 6.1.1), a certain basic trust was placed in the chief physician, as can be seen in the following statements in connection with the murder of Polish and Russian forced labourers in the asylum (for these patients specifically, see Sect. 7.1):

Q: Did you presume that all those Russians and Poles were incurably ill?

A: Yes.

Q: Why did you presume that?

A: [...] I had the opportunity to ask one who understood German if he was ill, and he said "Yes" and pointed to his lungs. I asked him if he was very ill, and he said that he

---

[4] It can be assumed that not only the gas murder phase contributed to this normalization effect, but that parts of the personnel had already gained further learning and socialization experiences in this respect in one of the actions in the meantime, but especially in the context of the detachment to Eichberg or Weilmünster (see Sects. 4.1 and 4.2) – where the killing methods were almost identical. For a more accurate reappraisal, however, one would have to be able to describe much more precisely which persons were active where, when and how.

had already been unable to work for six months. As a general rule I know this because I saw many diagnoses of the doctors.

Q: Did anyone tell you that all those who came there were incurably ill?

A: Yes; Bernotat told us that through Klein.

Q: Was there any chance of you determining how ill those people were?

A: I can't do that because I am not a doctor. (statement Ruoff, nursing staff, quoted from Kintner 1948, p. 178)

Q: Did you think that all these Russians and Poles were incurable?

A: I assumed that if the German doctors examined them they were reliable and that there was no doubt as to their testimony. (statement Willig, nursing staff, quoted after Kintner 1948, p. 185)

I thought it was assumed by a nurse that she followed all orders that were given to her. (statement Gumbmann, nursing staff, quoted from Kintner 1948, p. 143)

In this respect, a contradiction or even resistance to the instructions given by the doctors was not to be expected (HHStA/b, p. 28; see also Wettlaufer 1996, p. 307). In fact, without exception, all of the defendants belonging to the nursing staff at the Hadamar trial pointed out at the general meeting that they had been active primarily in view of the instructions emanating from the doctors (HHStA/b, p. 28).

Moreover, in the second phase of the murders, but also among the nursing staff themselves, much more emphasis was placed on a multi-level hierarchy system in the institution, which led to an even more insistent diffusion or delegation of responsibility. The distribution of command as well as decision-making processes and the accompanying responsibility for deeds could thus be spread over significantly more places (Welzer 2005, p. 120.). The head nurse Huber pointed out in this context, for example, that although the medication murders were indeed a crime to be condemned, her own activity was exempt from this insofar as her tasks had already been exhausted in the previous conference, the (pre-)selection of the sick and the passing on of notes (Wettlaufer 1996, pp. 326, 329):

I gave the note to the ward sister. What she did, I don't know. Only the names were on it. The medicine, that had already been discussed, that was a general discussion, and that's where it stayed. Now what the night stand was actually supposed to give? I don't know. (statement Huber, nursing staff, HHStA/a, p. 80)

My part in the elimination of patients now consisted in the fact that, knowing what was going on, I handed over the ward nurse's notes to Dr. Wahlmann and passed on his instructions in writing to the other nurses. This was my participation, which I also regard as guilt and must impute to myself. In contrast, in not a single case did I myself

carry out a killing or suggest a patient to Dr. Wahlmann for disposal. (statement
Huber, nursing staff, quoted after Wettlaufer 1996, p. 329)

The partialization of responsibility demonstrated here by Huber continued among
the hierarchically lower ranking ward nurses, in that, for example (but of course not
exclusively), it was emphasized that they themselves had administered the intended
drugs to only comparatively few persons (statement Reuter, nursing staff, HHStA/a,
p. 68), deliberately administering such low doses that the patients could not have
died from them under normal circumstances (statement by L. Thomas, nursing
staff, HHStA/a, p. 60; statement by Zielke, nursing staff, HHStA/a, p. 98), and/or
that the murders had to be carried out solely at the behest of the head nurses or the
doctor (statement by Gumbmann, nursing staff, quoted from Benedict 2003, p. 73;
statement by L. Thomas, nursing staff, HHStA/a, p. 60). This diffusion of responsibility can also be exemplified by the nurse Lückoff:

A: I only gave sleeping pills when they were loud and in the form I was taught. [...]

Q: Were there people dead the other morning?

A: No. Of those I have given medication to, not once have any of them been dead the
other morning. I also gave injections, [...]. These people were still asleep in the morning. [...] Willich injected people afterwards. I knew that I had to do preliminary work.
I did this preliminary work because I was forced to after all. [...] These patients were
so undernourished that even two tablets had an effect, so that they were still asleep in
the morning. The patients received the injections at midnight and when they were
asleep. The dose was never so great as to cause death. That someone else would still
give something was clear to me. (statement Lückoff, nursing staff, HHStA/a, p. 89)

One's own participation could thus always be seen as "something else" (Welzer
2005, p. 142), so that "the specific execution of the deed in each case was always
[considered] more "humane" than the "more inhumane" of the others" (ibid.).
Above all, no one had to feel responsible or guilty for the "big picture" under these
circumstances (Sandner 2003, p. 707).

In this context, it is also striking that the described, supposedly gentle or protective ways of acting of the nursing staff, all have in common that they never resulted
in loud resistance. Instead, the work – which was undoubtedly unpleasant for the
perpetrators – could be carried out better or worse, so that the instructions were
ultimately followed regardless and the correctness of the deeds was never questioned publicly or aloud (Welzer 2005, p. 203). So even if, as in Lückoff's case (see
above), lower dosages were indeed deliberately dispensed, this in itself did not
matter at all, because even such supposed deviations were perfectly compatible
with the institution's internal medical method of liquidation. Lückoff himself was

obviously aware of this, which is clear from the fact that he spoke of the *preliminary work* to be completed.

Finally, another mechanism that relieved responsibility was at the root of the starvation deaths, which have received comparatively less detailed attention in this work: In Hadamar, the deprivation of food was indeed a targeted method of murder, but in this case induced not by the nursing staff, but by the more senior officials of the District Association as well as the administrative officer of the asylum (Sandner 2003, pp. 589ff., 700f.; see also Schmidt-von Blittersdorff et al. 1996, p. 110f., who show that Klein "corrected" the food supplies for the worse for the patients). Meanwhile, the Hadamar nursing staff may have come to the conclusion that the food rations provided were "determined in view of allocations of a higher order" (statement by Huber, nursing staff, cited in Sandner 2003, p. 589), but all in all it was difficult to trace the responsibilities for this (ibid., p. 591ff.). Presumably, however, it was no coincidence that death by starvation, as the method of murder that could not be subordinated to the medical method of liquidation described, represented a contextual condition that was apparently hardly or even uninfluenceable for the nursing staff, while at the same time it was precisely through this that the image of the emaciated, disease-prone and ultimately "unworthy of life" psychiatric patients could be emphatically plausibilized (similarly Schmidt-von Blittersdorff et al. 1996, p. 111): "These people were already half-starved and so weakened that I had the conviction that death meant salvation for them. I knew that the drugs had a lethal effect" (statement by Reuter, nursing staff, quoted from Kneuker and Steglich 1985, p. 29).

6.1.5   The Cycle of Killings

In addition to the known or remembered selection criteria described so far on the one hand (6.1.2) and the direct instructions on the other (6.1.4), there was a third central trigger for the murders in the asylum, as a glance at the asylum occupancy rate and the death rate (which ran parallel) makes clear (Schmidt-von Blittersdorff et al. 1996, p. 108f.): Murders increased considerably after the arrival of several or larger transports and the resulting (over-)occupancy of the asylum (Faulstich 1998, p. 548; also Sandner 2003, p. 595). The number of killings thus did not settle at a constant or arbitrary value, but instead varied, as did the transports themselves, according to "need", i.e. according to the occupancy rate of the institution as well as possible upcoming transports (Sandner 2003, p. 648; Schmidt-von Blittersdorff et al. 1996, p. 115; also Faulstich 1998, pp. 305, 621).

From the perspective of the nursing staff, this created a veritable "vicious circle" (Masuch 1985): as soon as overcrowding occurred, the need to kill increased in order to restore sufficient capacity in the asylum. However, the killings carried out in this context simultaneously created new space for further deliveries of patients. In this context, the Nassau District Association issued a quasi-continuous guarantee for the (new) admission of sick people, which could only be maintained if the occupancy of the asylum would be "reduced" accordingly on a regular basis (Sandner 2006, p. 150). At the same time, the Berlin authorities ensured that regular transports of (mostly foreign) patients actually took place (George 2006, p. 236; Sandner 2003, pp. 648, 653, 701). For example, in a letter to the Reich Commissioner for state hospitals and nursing homes, Bernotat calculated that it would take 2–3 weeks to have about 100 patients murdered in Hadamar, only to be able to receive 100 new patients as a result (Sandner 2003, p. 638f.).[5]

In this way, the need to murder the sick developed again and again – especially since the second central contextual condition of the killings, the Allied air bombardments (Chap. 5), became increasingly aggravated as time went on (Faulstich 1998, p. 312f.). The administrative superiors Bernotat and Klein, in particular, accordingly demanded widespread killings when new mass transfers to Hessen-Nassau were imminent (Sandner 2003, p. 648; Süß 2003, p. 353). Conversely, two nurses commented that "the stock was always replenished" (statement by Kneissler, nursing staff, cited in Sandner 2003, p. 648) when "a larger number of beds were free again" (statement by Hackbarth, nursing staff, ibid.).

---

[5] Financially, this agreement was associated with advantages for the District Association because, on the one hand, Hadamar predominantly admitted out-of-town patients. An own contribution to the financing of care costs was not necessary here (George 2006, p. 235f.). Accordingly, the transports to Hadamar described above (see Chap. 5) were made up of almost 90% external patients (Sandner 2003, p. 649, 2006, p. 150) – which, incidentally, is a further, very clear indication of the function of the Hadamar LHA as a *central* murder institution (Chap. 5). Secondly, as we have already seen, most of the patients admitted in this framework were not killed immediately after their arrival, but only after the patients' stay had exceeded a certain duration (which varied according to the individual) and had thus brought in corresponding care funds and labour (Sandner 2003, p. 701). The large number of out-of-town patients was therefore financially advantageous for the District Association from two perspectives. The worse the people were accommodated, the greater the economic benefit (ibid., pp. 648, 701) – which in turn can be traced back to the administrative method of starvation. Economically, this system of transports and responsive killings remained advantageous primarily because permanent patient replacements from institutions outside the district could be guaranteed as a result of the air raids happening all over Germany (Lilienthal 2010, p. 108).

6.1.6   Lack of Exit Options

With regard to the possible exit options, the Hadamar cadre held two conflicting basic positions (Wettlaufer 1996, p. 314): One (smaller) grouping pointed out that a resignation had been possible in principle, but that the exit could not or would not have been made for various reasons – one of which, for example, would have been the difficult economic and social situation that a loss of employment would have entailed (for this, see also Sect. 3.2.3) (for example, statement by Bellin, nursing staff, Kintner 1948, p. 139). The rest of the collective, meanwhile, pointed out that an exit would not have been possible at all (Wettlaufer 1996, p. 314). Precisely, it was the fear of a concentration camp or the death penalty that had a corresponding effect on the latter grouping, because both of these potential sanctions were hardly perceived as a realistic option for action:

> Q: Did you actually fear that you were going to a concentration camp if you attempted to leave there?
>
> Huber: Yes, certainly I would have gotten there.
>
> [...]
>
> Q: But what you are trying to tell us is that you would have gone to a concentration camp if you had attempted to leave?
>
> Huber: Yes, I was afraid of that, and that would have been a certainty.
>
> [...]
>
> Q: You did decide to stay there at this place where Russian and Polish people were being murdered in lieu of going to a concentration camp, did you not?
>
> Huber: Who wants to go to a concentration camp? I was afraid of that too. (statement by Huber, nursing staff, quoted from Kintner 1948, p. 119f.)

Similarly, Nurse L. Thomas pointed out that although she found the medical orders issued to her terrible, she was unable to defend herself against them because she would have been too afraid of the consequences: "For sure I would have ended up in a concentration camp, I believe that for sure" (nursing staff, HHStA/a, p. 60f.). This concern was also expressed openly by other employees, for example by the nurses Kneissler (nursing staff, Wettlaufer 1996, p. 314), Schrankel (nursing staff, HHStA/a, p. 407) or Weimer:

> Q: What do you think would have happened to that person if he had said, I'm not going to do that, I refuse to do that? I simply cannot do that out of inner conviction?

A: According to my imagination, they would have been sent to a concentration camp. After all, I had already allowed myself to lose my nerve and I was shown who dictates here and who is in charge. Since I did not want to commit suicide, I complied. (statement Weimer, nursing staff, HHStA/a, p. 111)

Despite this, however, the court was unable to establish an actual state of coercion – coercion to participate could only be proven in the case of the personnel who were obliged to serve (Friedlander 1997, p. 378ff.; Meusch 2006, p. 314). This was mainly due to the fact that some of the personnel admitted that there had never been any openly communicated threats regarding a possible stay in a concentration camp. So all in all, on the one hand, the concerns in this regard were rather due to the general interpretations of the situation (see, for example, Willig's statement, nursing staff, Kintner 1948, p. 82). But on the other hand, the staff was also aware of cases in which former employees had had to serve longer sentences – including a stay in a concentration camp (for examples, see the statements of the sisters Huber, Bellin, Zachow, Hackbarth and Gumbmann, nursing staff, Kintner 1948, pp. 118 et seq, 128, 138ff; also Sandner 2003, pp. 477f., 647). The staff thus found themselves in a rather ambivalent situation as far as the possibility of leaving was concerned.

During the time in which the murders were practiced in Hadamar, some attempts to resign or to leave the organization can be ascertained. In general, however, it was true that such efforts through formal and official channels were almost exclusively in vain (see, for example, Bacher's statement, office staff, HHStA/a, p. 148; statement J. Thomas, office staff, HHStA/a, p. 129). In particular, head nurse Huber issued several dismissals, all of which were rejected by Klein and/or Bernotat (see, in addition to her own statements in this regard, corroborating witness reports, for example HHStA/a, pp. 48, 51, 73, 227, 407). At a later point in time, her request to leave Hadamar was even rejected by Dr. Wahlmann in the first instance, since, according to the statements of the chief physician, the tasks to be performed had to be done and they could not avoid them (statement Huber, nursing staff, HHStA/a, p. 50).

The actual possibilities to withdraw from service in Hadamar in the medium to long term, if necessary even permanently, are to be differentiated above all according to gender-specific aspects. In addition to that, a correspondingly intensive illness was another valid reason to leave the institution. Such was the case for Pauline Kneissler, who did not return to Hadamar after a longer period of illness (statement Huber, nursing staff, Kintner 1948, p. 129; similarly the case of Olga U., Wettlaufer

1996, p. 312)[6]. The gender-specific aspects manifest themselves in the fact that women had the option of at least temporarily resigning from service due to pregnancy (Wettlaufer 1996, p. 311). In a few cases, female employees did not have to return to the institution at all after giving birth – this included, for example, Sisters Korsch and Schrankel (statement Schrankel, nursing staff, HHStA/a, p. 79; statement Huber, nursing staff, Kintner 1948, p. 129; HHStA/b, p. 39). Meanwhile, Nurse Weimer was able to force her exit by feigning pregnancy (HHStA/a, p. 105; HHStA/b, pp. 22, 39).

However, even pregnancy was no guarantee of leave. Thus, although the employee Judith S. gave birth to a child in 1943, she still lived in the LHA Hadamar and continued to help out in the office even beyond the end of the war (Sandner 2003, p. 621). J. Thomas, meanwhile, described:

> I said I was expecting a child. Bernotat then said that was no reason to stop working. In 1943 I tried again, after the child was born. Bernotat told me personally that I could only be dismissed after an examination by his personal physician [...]. This Dr. Koch examined me in Oct. 1943 and declared me fully fit for work. (office staff, HHStA/a, p. 129f.)

The alternative for male nurses was to enlist in the Wehrmacht (Hoffmann 2010, p. 254f.) – an option that was certainly not all that attractive from their perspective (see, for example, Friedlander 1997, p. 376; more generally also Gruber 2015, p. 38f.). By the end of March,1943, 15 male employees had been called up for military service (Sandner 2003, p. 617f.; Schmidt-von Blittersdorff et al. 1996, p. 111; also Wettlaufer 1996, p. 312). But in spite of the growing military need, it can also be questioned whether a personally initiated draft amounted to a legitimate and actually available exit option (see, for example, the statement Ruoffs, nursing staff, Kintner 1948, p. 178f.; statement Lindner, office staff, HHStA/a, p. 124). In the final verdict of the Hadamar trial, for example, it is stated that it

---

[6] Pauline Kneissler was instead – which was not established by the American military court – seconded to the Kaufbeuren asylum in Irsee from April 1944 because the asylum director there, Valentin Faltlhauser, had "requested forces from Berlin for the express purpose of killing the mentally ill [...]" (Schmidt et al. 2012, p. 291; see also Mitscherlich and Mielke 1995, p. 243). To all appearances, no "euthanasia" had taken place in the Bavarian asylum up to this point (Schmidt et al. 2012, p. 292). After the involvement of Kneissler, however, about 254 patients died on her ward by the end of the war, while the remaining five women's wards had only nine deaths in the same period – and these were due to (verifiable) infectious diseases (ibid.). This example once again makes it quite clear what a significant role prior experience and normalized (killing) expectations (6.1.2 and 6.1.3) played in the implementation of the deeds.

would have been quite possible for the orderly Reuter to get out of the institution if he had enlisted in the Wehrmacht (HHStA/b, p. 45). Reuter himself, on the other hand, reports on these facts as follows:

> Then, in the time up to the middle of September, I once expressed the wish to Mr. Klein that he would like to transfer me to Schnepfenhausen, that I would only dream of naked corpses at night, and then he said: Yes, if that no longer suits you, if you no longer want that, then I must report you to the military. [...] That's when I got the order to report for duty, on 5.10.42 in Wetzlar. Then I went to Mr. Klein, and he screamed and raved, no, there's no way! I can't hand you over! Who else is to bury the people! Then he immediately telephoned Wiesbaden. I then went out. Later he asked for me and said: Reuter, you stay here! For now. I spoke to Wiesbaden, you will not go to Wetzler until Wiesbaden has given you the word. On 4.10.42 in the morning I went to Mr. Klein and told him that I was leaving for home at two o'clock this afternoon, that no decision had been received yet, and that I had to be in Wetzlar tomorrow morning at nine o'clock. His response: You stay here. I had to stay there. I said: well, if I don't get a decision, you'll have to take responsibility. And in the afternoon at 5 o'clock my wife called me and told me that a card had come from Wetzlar, that I had been deferred from the service, and that I should send back the draft notice immediately. So I nevertheless remained in Hadamar until February 3. On 3 February 1943 I had to report to the military again, joined the Landesschützen in Krakow, there I remained in the military until the end of the war. (statement by Reuter, nursing staff, HHStA/a, p. 67)

With a view on the departures that actually took place, it can thus be stated that the employees could theoretically withdraw from their duties, but the practical implementation of this was enormously problematic. In particular, nursing staff who killed the sick probably found it comparatively difficult to leave their jobs permanently, because it was more difficult to find a suitable replacement for them (Sandner 2003, p. 617f.; this is also indicated by the findings in Sect. 6.1.3). In any case, it is also true that the leading (administrative) forces in Hadamar left open the possibility of temporarily or (very rarely) permanently dismissing staff from service in individual cases in principle – as in the case of Sister Edit Korsch, who was dismissed from service not only because of her pregnancy but also because of incidents of "indiscipline" (Sandner 2003, p. 621). As was the case with the recruitment measures, then, a certain level of agreement with and conviction of the eugenic campaign seems to have played a role in determining a possible dismissal attempt, in addition to political loyalty. What is striking at this point is once again that all concessions were made in silence, i.e. even the possible forms of resignation (illness, resignation or compulsory military service) were at best latent forms of resistance, thus in the end never questioning the legitimacy or legality of the formal killing expectations.

6.2   Maintained Knowledge Structures and Continued (Interactional) Experiences

A more detailed look at the medication killings in Hadamar (Sects. 6.1–6.1.6) shows that these were by no means indiscriminate or wildly carried out mass killings. In addition to the change in central contextual conditions – meaning the air war and starvation –, a number of organisationally supported patterns can be observed in the second murder phase, which in their combination made the practices possible or at least facilitated them. These include the medical primacy underlying the killings (Sect. 6.1.1), the hierarchization of the patients within the institution (Sect. 6.1.2), a staff that was in principle already familiar with the campaign and its actions (Sect. 6.1.3), the extensive (hierarchically legitimized) diffusion or delegation of responsibility (Sect. 6.1.4), a regularly repeated cycle between the killings and the subsequent new patient transports (Sect. 6.1.5) and the lack of exit options for the staff (Sect. 6.1.6).

Despite all the changes and modifications, it is unquestionable that, from the perspective of the Hadamar cadre, the situation was not completely different or even contrary: supposedly lethally sick patients were still murdered under the pretext of mercy killing, or, from the staff's point of view, were to be "euthanized" on the basis of a medically diagnosed necessity. In this respect, there is no doubt that the entire staff was aware within a short period of time of what had to happen in the asylum (Sandner 2003, p. 622f.). These fundamental similarities in organizational expectations as well as actual actions was crucial for the implementation of the new murder practices in the second phase:

> What the purpose of the tablets was, no one told me that directly. I guess one could hear what was going on. Not much was said about it because other work was given to us. It was a matter of course that these patients were to be killed. It was known everywhere throughout. And that these tablets were used for this purpose was clear to me. (statement by Moos, nursing staff, HHStA/a, p. 93f.)

> Q: Did these slips of paper that were passed around bear the signature of a doctor? Or was there anything outwardly recognizable to the nurses that that was approved by the doctor?

> A: I took a simple piece of paper. I wrote down the names that the doctor gave. I passed the piece of paper on. Signed by the doctor? No. I did that in the presence of the doctor.

> Q: How could the nurses tell from a mere list of names what to do with these slips of paper?

> A: They knew that; it was common.

Q: Who told the nurses that they were to be euthanized based on these notes?

A: They knew that. The nurses came from Berlin and then it was arranged. The doctor ordered that he would be responsible for the patients he determined, and I was to make a note of them, and I passed this on to the nurses. (statement by Huber, nursing staff, HHStA/a, p. 78f.)

It should not be ruled out, for example, that there were greater inhibitions because of the more personal method of killing. What is decisive, however, is that the killings in the period from 1942 onwards could also be subordinated to the previously customary behaviour patterns and expectations. The actors oriented themselves to familiar, *normalized* behaviors that had already been institutionalized, rationalized, and socialized (Sects. 3.1–3.3) in order to cope with the divergent method of killing through subsequent *"sense making"* (Ashforth and Fried 1988, p. 308, emphasis added; Gioia 1992, pp. 386, 388). In this context, similar to what was noted at the beginning about the institutionalization of the practices (Sect. 3.1), the implementation of the acts was never dependent on a moral or ethical endorsement. In the end, it did not matter how the acting personnel, far removed from their organisational role, thought about the killings, because in the organisationally determined process such an ethical dimension was not even envisaged or of importance (Gioia 1992, pp. 379f., 385; also Welzer 2005, p. 117).

In many cases, therefore, it was not necessary to provide more detailed or generally applicable instructions or briefings to the staff with regard to the tasks to be performed (see, for example, the statements of J. Thomas, office staff, HHStA/a, p. 131; Moos, nursing staff, HHStA/a, p. 101). Those involved were already clear about what had to happen. In this respect, there was talk within the institution of a "second action", which was basically to follow the same goals that had already been issued at the time of the gas murders (Sandner 2003, p. 622):

Q: Now what thoughts did he (Wahlmann) have about that, if he didn't inform the sister about what happens if the sister is not legitimate?

A: It was self-evident that the head nurse knew about it! Where did she get her legitimation from? The foundation matters – that had already been done before, the nurses had done that too. That was a matter of course. (statement by Wahlmann, chief physician, HHStA/a, p. 39)

What was done before with gassing was now continued in a different form. We were also told this by Klein. Klein reminded us that we had to do the same as with the foundation. The institution had exactly the same purpose, only the form was different. (statement by Moos, nursing staff, HHStA/a, p. 94)

That's when a colleague came to me and said the same action was going on, but in a different form. She also said that I was destined to do it. [...] I knew that I was assigned to continue the campaign in Hadamar. (statement Zielke, nursing staff, HHStA/a, p. 97f.)

A significant part of the explanation of the medication killings thus lies, according to my proposed interpretation derived from the explanations, in the continuation of previous knowledge and practices as well as the accompanying preserved interpretations of the personnel – a personnel that was already familiar with the events of the National Socialist euthanasia in the broader sense, its notion of "life unworthy of life", as well as the widely developed and institutionalized willingness to obey the organizational structures. The events in the second phase allow the conclusion that the killings are based, on the one hand, on *knowledge structures* held in memory, i.e. based above all on the former institutionalization as well as the rationalization of the deeds (Sects. 3.1 and 3.2). On the other hand, *continued interactional experiences* also play a central role, which resembles a continuity of the pillar of socialisation (Sect. 3.3). The acts thus ultimately appear suitable to the actors because they lay within their regular horizon of expectations (Kühl 2014a, p. 277), i.e. from a subjective (the perpetrator's) point of view, these were situations that they had already encountered in such or at least a similar way in the context of their membership role (Ashforth and Fried 1988, p. 309f.; Gioia 1992, p. 385; Gioia and Poole 1984, p. 450f.; also Welzer 2005, p. 46).

Therefore, in the second phase, an action structure is found that has enabled the personnel to complete the killing task assigned to them together, i.e. within and in the sense of the organisational setting (Welzer 2005, p. 131). Those acting on the spot have no doubts about the relevance and correctness of their deeds (ibid., p. 216; further Bandura 1990, p. 30). In this sense, they were not unstructured actions or actions based on chance, but practices that were in line with a clear organisational agenda underlying the acts, in which a (pre-)determined reaction – namely the killing process in the institution – was set off as soon as a corresponding trigger occurred (Klatetzki 2015, p. 156; Kühl 2014a, p. 282f.). The scheme or organisational *script* described for the killings (Gioia 1992; Klatetzki 2015, p. 156f.) can be depicted as follows (Fig. 6.1).

This constantly repeating congruent sequence of events, beginning with the arrival of the transports and the subsequent killings within a medical primate, which, in addition to episodes of nursing normality, included the hierarchization of the sick based on an apparently medical basis as well as the medical method of liquidation, led to the death of the patients, whereupon the bureaucratic post-processing began.

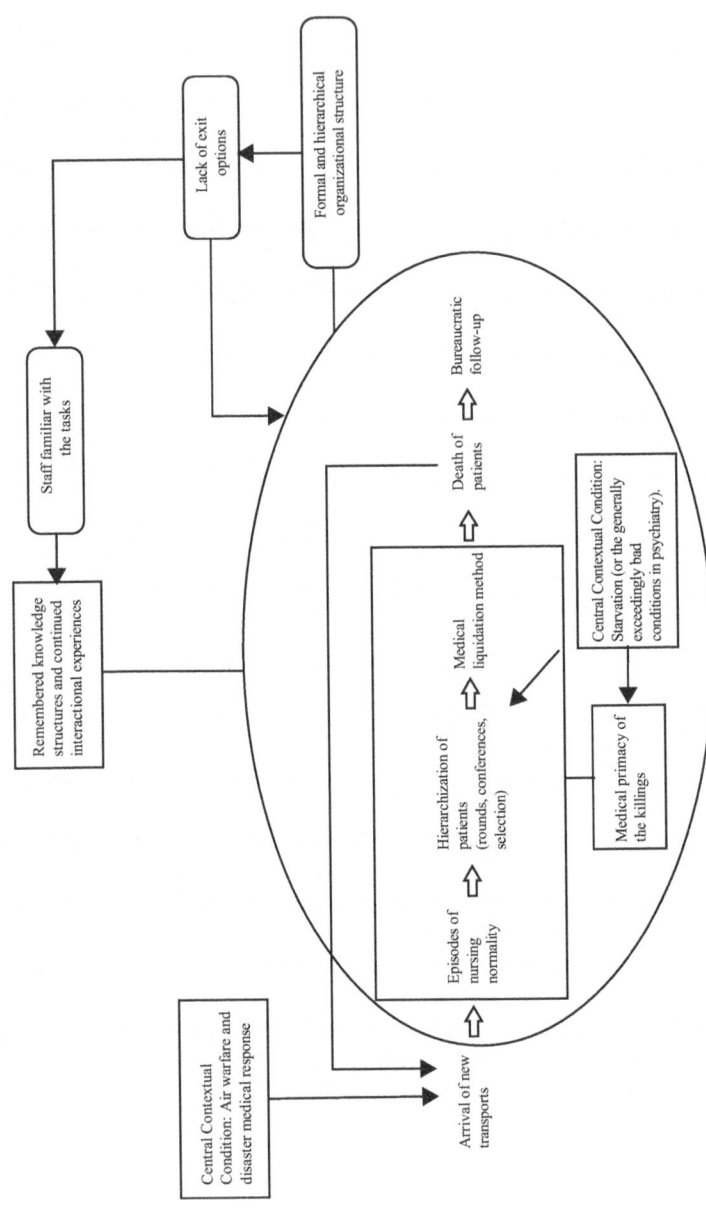

Fig. 6.1 The killing scheme of the second phase

There were two central contextual conditions that had a direct impact on this process: First, there was the comparatively briefly treated starvation or the exceedingly poor conditions in psychiatric hospitals in general, which in a number of cases not to be underestimated placed patients in conditions that, in accordance with National Socialist views, plausibilized a need for "mercy death" to be brought about. Secondly, the air war and the resulting medical emergency management of the regime (especially in the persona of Brandt and Linden; see Chap. 5) should be emphasized. The continuous arrival of patients from the areas threatened by the bombings or already hit by them, as well as the internal exitus of the sick in the institution that reacted to or depended on this, set the cycle of medication murders in the Hadamar killing centre in motion again and again.

In the meantime, this routine and regular pattern has remained so stable over a long period of time,[7] precisely because it was carried out by employees who had already been largely familiar with the tasks (and in this respect could fall back on their remembered knowledge structures or interpretations as well as their interactional experiences made up to that point), the exit options made it hardly possible to get out of this cycle, and finally, or quite especially, because the murder programme was carried out within the framework of a formally secured, strictly hierarchical organisational structure. The killings were thus *only* legitimate if they were carried out, on the one hand, in the sense of the medical primate and, on the other hand, within the framework of the organisational membership role or organisational structure (see also Sect. 3.2.3) – which, in conclusion, can be subsumed as a clear indication that the second phase of murder in Hadamar was also not only about organised, but in addition, about *normalized* brutalities. These were provided with a regulated beginning, middle and end (Welzer 2005, p. 14, 147).

---

[7] The scheme described here, and thus the murders in general, famously came to a halt only after it was broken off by an external force (in the form of the American military troops). It can be assumed that the cycle or scheme could have remained active for a (much) longer time, especially under wartime conditions (Sandner 2003, p. 648).

Conclusion: The Normalization of Organized Brutalities

Organizational sociology devotes comparatively little attention to issues that, due to their unprecedented brutality, are perceived as central ruptures of modern society (Kühl 2005, p. 90; further Friedrich 2012, p. 2f.). There does not seem to be an obvious reason for this. In any case, the results of the present study suggest that regular societal monstrosities can also be explained – at least in part – with exceedingly regular approaches that have been familiar to organizational sociology for a long time (Chap. 2). In doing so, the position elaborated here was able to show how a multitude of individuals, who were by no means trained or otherwise predisposed to mass murder, could engage in precisely such acts in a common and always regulated manner. Various organisational mechanisms and techniques helped to institutionalise the illegal acts in a first step, i.e. above all to create a routine intended for this purpose (Sect. 3.1). The practices were also rationalized, which not only legitimised them but often even made them appear highly desirable (Sect. 3.2). Finally, deliberately selected members were introduced to the processes in such a way that rapid familiarisation and widespread acceptance of the deviant practices could be achieved relatively effortlessly and without difficulty (Sect. 3.3). As a result of this *normalization* of expectations and actions, the employees characterized their activities as indifferent – in other words, they ultimately took them for granted and did not openly question them. The fact that these behaviors could even be maintained in a modified way after some central conditions and characteristics of the processes had changed (Chaps. 4, 5, 6) is to a significant extent due to the fact that the staff, familiar with the tasks in the broadest sense, still working within the framework of a well known and established formal-hierarchical organizational structure, could fall back on previous, already socialized interactional experiences and on knowledge structures or interpretations about the apparently medically

D. Firkus, *On the Normalization of Organized Brutalities*, https://doi.org/10.1007/978-3-658-41515-0_7

necessary, therefore justified euthanasia. The resulting action structure was solidified by two additional contextual conditions as well as a lack of exit options. How stable this killing scheme (Fig. 6.1) actually was becomes apparent in the fact that only an external (to be precise: a military) force was able to bring it to a final halt (Sects. 6.1.1–6.2).

In the course of this work, it should have become clear that research in the sociology of organizations can offer a thoroughly fruitful and compatible perspective in such a context (see also Sect. 7.1). Despite all the plausibilities that have been sketched out in this framework, however, the study is not intended to call for an all-encompassing organizational sociology that henceforth attempts to identify possible organizational mechanisms for explaining all brutalities or violent acts. Insofar as I have already not indulged in the *deflationary* tendencies of the concept of organization in this contribution (Chap. 2), I cannot and will likewise not submit to the fate of *inflationary,* often self-overestimating contributions within the sociology of organizations (Tacke 2015, p. 278f.). There are plenty of examples for contrary assumptions – one might think of, for instance, studies on so-called "school shootings" (Braun 2016; Katz 2016), the almost daily conflicts in marriages (Collins 2011, p. 202ff.) or the spontaneously emerging violent activities in protests (Nassauer 2016), in which organizational sociological analyses would be anything but meaningful.

Organized brutalities that assume such a scale as National Socialist euthanasia may certainly not be explicable solely through a genuinely organizational sociological perspective. Particularly with regard to the Third Reich, there are ultimately too many individual and specific historical features to which a section of sociology alone cannot pay sufficient tribute (Katz 1993, p. 14; Kühl 2014a, p. 325f.). But at the same time, it is true that an attempt to explain such a social phenomenon is and remains incomplete without a fundamental understanding of the social system based on memberships, which can induce or assure conformity of action even in the face of exceedingly far-reaching demands (Chap. 2). After all, as has been shown, it is no coincidence that the many untrained individuals – irrespective of the respective killing phase – only developed and maintained obedience as well as the willingness to participate in the atrocities within the framework of their organizational membership, while at the same time discarding this docility outside of their membership role.

At the beginning of this project, I pointed out that from a sociological point of view, there are no reasons whatsoever for not dealing with events from the period of National Socialism (Sect. 1.2). On the contrary, there is even the suggestion that it is precisely the adoption of such an analytical position that is able to highlight the potentials of an organizational sociological perspective (Kühl 2005, p. 90f.). Not least, the analysis undertaken of the National Socialist murders of the sick themselves plausibilizes this assumption. In this context, however, it should be pointed out that the explanations were at no time based on an attempt to trivialise or even justify the acts in any way. Researchers dealing with such atrocities may indeed produce formulations, perspectives or even results that do not seem obvious at first, and may even be perceived as unpleasant by a certain readership or audience (Katz 1993, p. 4; on this problematization, see also Chap. 1 and Sect. 1.1). But neither the present work nor – bearing in mind the necessary caution that such generalizations usually require – other thematic discussions of the mass murders carried out during the Nazi regime (or elsewhere) can or will engage in such trivialization or justification. Sociological discussions of topics such as euthanasia and the "extermination of life unworthy of life" can only help us to better understand these atrocities. But they cannot, do not want to, and should not cast them in a proper light.

7.1 Research Perspective(S): The Analytical Generality of the Elaborated Theses

In the context of this study, I have introduced an organizational sociological perspective into the context of National Socialist eugenic campaign that has received little or no attention to date. The assumptions and findings elaborated in the course of the paper were thereby primarily case-related and thus initially the result of an investigation focused on the Hadamar asylum. However, this does not rule out the "analytical generality" of the argument beyond the reference case (Hoebel 2018, p. 177), i.e. that the notion of the normalization of organized brutalities can be applied in a very similar way to other euthanasia institutions as well. The elaborated explanatory approach is thus (ideally) characterized by the property of being transferable to further empirical cases as well as to subsequent theoretical preferences thanks to its abstractly formulated premises and principles (Aljets and Hoebel 2017, p. 7; also Kühl 2014a, p. 325f., 2018/2019, p. 121).

One can certainly raise the justified objection that a comprehensive analytical generality cannot be achieved, or can only be achieved with difficulty, because this is solely a detailed individual case study. While this is true, it does not preclude the possibility of obtaining reliable information regarding a broader social phenomenon (Flyvbjerg 2006). The mechanisms and structures elaborated centrally in the course of the article can certainly be understood as a heuristic-analytical handout that would be of great use as a "method of discovery" (Abbott 2004) for subsequent analyses of other euthanasia institutions. The context-dependent knowledge gained from the reference case could function, at least in places, as generalized context-independent knowledge (Flyvbjerg 2006, p. 221ff.).

In this sense, the claim to analytical generality in connection with the events of the first murder phase seem to be extremely plausible at first glance in view of the basically similar processes within the asylums. Ultimately, the functioning of the six gas murder institutions differed at most marginally from one another in many facets (Sandner 2003, pp. 487, 703; see also Sect. 1.2; for the Hartheim institution, see Kepplinger 2008).[1] This was already indicated in the analytical discussion (Chap. 3) insofar as in some places references were made not only explicitly to Hadamar, but also to events from other or all asylums. This already provided first indications of the validity, reliability and, not least, objectivity of the research pro-gramme used here, as well as its possible analytical generality – aspects that are usually criticised in individual case studies with regard to their "generalisability" (Flyvbjerg 2006, p. 221).

Of course, it cannot be assumed that the analytical three-step process described for the normalization of practices on the one hand (Chap. 3) and the killing scheme identified for the second phase on the other (Chap. 6) can be transferred one-to-one to other cases. Rather, it is to be expected that there will be minor variations in the analysis of other asylums or asylum killings, so some steps may be skipped, merged, or even replaced altogether. However, this is due less to a contradiction than to the result of social reality – especially since the conceptions, together with the associated strands of argumentation, are designed and formulated to be open or flexible enough to take account of any modifications and at the same time to be able to incorporate and subordinate them to the underlying pattern (Klatetzki 2015, p. 157; also Gioia 1992, p. 385f.; Gioia and Poole 1984, pp. 450, 452).

Especially for the second murder phase, however, it would have to be clarified much more precisely in a previous step for whom or what exactly such an analytical generality would be plausible. This already begins with the question of whether the elaborated killing scheme can also be made valid in this (or a similar) form for the expanded spectrum of murder victims that can be found in Hadamar with in-creasing time (see, for example, Faulstich 1998, p. 546; Lilienthal 2006a, p. 171; Sandner 2003, p. 654, 2006, p. 151). Particularly noteworthy is the comparatively large number of approximately 400–500 Polish and Russian forced laborers who were considered *unfit for work* due to infectious diseases – mostly tuberculosis –

---

[1] The overlaps are partly quite astonishing. In the analysis of the gas murders I referred, among other things, to the celebrated dehumanization of the 10,000 corpse in Hadamar (Sect. 3.2.4). We can detect a very similar celebration in the Grafeneck asylum, for example, where, to all appearances, a brass band was also on site (Klee 1986, p. 119).

and were therefore dismissed from their original employment (Friedlander 1997, p. 265; Kaufmann and Schulmeyer 1996; Koessler 1953, p. 740f.). In this context, it seems reasonable to assume that the Hadamar killing schema served as a prop for the staff – just as the remembered knowledge structures for said schema itself originally did – so that the new situations and expectations created by the organization (i.e., the killing of the forced laborers) could be managed by drawing on fundamentally similar, older experiences they had already had in the context of their membership (Gioia and Poole 1984, pp. 449f., 453). One of many parallels (see, for example, Kaufmann and Schulmeyer 1996, p. 227ff.) lies in the renewed practice of medical liquidation, which was equally legitimized by a corresponding (apparent) medical necessity (on this also Kintner 1948, pp. 15f., 21; Koessler 1953, pp. 740, 743, 748):

> It was to be seen from these medical papers without a doubt that all sick people who arrived had been treated in hospitals for several months because of tuberculosis. [...] After I had seen that from the papers, that evening I myself went up to the ward and I myself saw a great part of these sick people after they were undressed. [...] In a large number of these diseased people, pus areas could be seen in the body the size of a hand. [...] I am of the sure conviction that if the gentlemen of the Commission had a chance to see such a transport it would not be difficult for them to judge whether the deeds which took place at Hadamar and whether this case can be looked upon as a violation of International Law. I myself believe it is cruel that such people who were incurable had to endure pain, if one would let them live longer, because this was a big danger to Eastern workers at that time" (statement Klein, head of the institution, quoted after Kintner 1948, p. 199f.).

> A: [...] we mostly gave tablets, and it was only in those cases when some of them did not want to take the tablets because they were bitter that we gave injections. [...]

> Q: But in this case of the 15 women in the room upstairs, was it syringes that were used at that time?

> A: Yes, because they were all women and they don't like to take tablets. [...] men just take those without any trouble. (statement Ruoff, nursing staff, quoted after Kintner 1948, p. 175f.).

A notable modification to the usual scheme, meanwhile, lies in the fact that the described episodes of nursing normality (see Sect. 6.1.1; Fig. 6.1) were given comparatively little prominence. For example, unlike the German patients, the forced labourers were in all cases killed on the day of their arrival (Kaufmann and Schulmeyer 1996, p. 277). Exactly why this variation became established cannot be definitively determined – was it, for example, in response to tuberculosis, which was portrayed as highly contagious (Friedlander 1997, p. 265f.; Kaufmann and Schulmeyer 1996, pp. 258, 265f.; Lilienthal 2010, p. 107)? Or was the military defeat and the resulting collapse of the regime already so foreseeable at this point – the first transport of forced laborers did not reach Hadamar until mid-1944, after all (Lilienthal 2010, p. 107) – that central figures of the District Association and/or the Central Office wanted to maximize the killings of as many people as possible who did not conform to their own racial doctrine? At the very least, for the murders of the forced laborers, the traceable chain of command can be drawn beyond Klein and Bernotat to Gauleiter Springer (Lilienthal 2010, p. 107; Süß 2007, p. 128): "[…] he [meaning Klein, DF] explained that Bernotat and Springer had ordered that these patients, just like the German patients, were to be put aside according to law" (statement Ruoff, nursing staff, quoted after Kintner 1948, p. 174f.). Further clarification of possible continuities and breaks among the foreign forced laborers with regard to the elaborated killing scheme requires additional elaboration.

Meanwhile, if one looks beyond the case of Hadamar, the notion of analytical generality of the present theses for the period after the demonstrative stop could first be tested with regard to such institutions, which are also described as "murder centers" of the second phase. As presented earlier (Chap. 5), one possible interpretation, and the one preferred here, is to understand Hadamar not only as one, but instead as the central killing institution of the medication murders (see also Faulstich 1998, p. 580 f.; Lilienthal 2006a, p. 169, 2010; Sandner 2006, p. 147f.). Meanwhile, the historical "special case" of Hadamar can, to all appearances, be compared structurally and temporally with another, possibly even second asylum: In all likelihood, the Meseritz-Obrawalde asylum forms a corresponding counterpart (Faulstich 1998, pp. 615, 619; Sandner 2003, pp. 607, 649f., 703; also Lilienthal 2010, p. 100f.).[2] Faulstich (1998, p. 545) notes further similarities at the Großschweidnitz asylum, although the mortality rates here were significantly lower (ibid., p. 506; see also Süß 2003, p. 352ff., who lists Großschweidnitz alongside Hadamar as a killing centre, but takes an ambivalent position on Meseritz-Obrawalde).

Of particular interest in this context, however, are the institutions that operated much more extensively or exclusively under regional measures (see Sect. 4.2; for an overview, see Süß 2007). In view of the elaborated killing scheme, it can be assumed that the two central contextual variables in particular take on a different significance – the air war, for example, loses relevance for historical reasons, while the starvation of the patients gains in importance, perhaps even becoming much more a part of the central killing program. The rest of the process – i.e. above all

---

[2] A quite astonishing parallel between these two institutions lies in the fact that (to all appearances *only*) these two institutions were not run by their respective chief physicians, but the de facto management was instead incumbent on the respective administrative officials – in Hadamar, that is Alfons Klein (Faulstich 1998, p. 615; Sandner 2003, p. 650).

the medical primacy of the killings, including the episodes of nursing normality, the hierarchizations or selections of the sick made according to their ability to work, and the subsequent medical method of liquidation – seems to be almost identical (this is at least suggested by the conditions in the Kaufbeuren asylum, see Schmidt et al. 2012, p. 287ff.; a parallel between the killing centers and Kaufbeuren is interestingly also found in Süß 2003, p. 354).

Whether and to what extent the scheme (Fig. 6.1) can be applied to such "regional asylums" is a question that needs to be examined empirically. It is quite conceivable that the elaborated killing scheme in this form is only plausible with regard to the "killing centres" of the second phase, while the "more freely" operating asylums are, all in all, subject to similar, yet divergent structures and mechanisms. The task of future sociological euthanasia research could thus also (or perhaps especially) lie in identifying different killing programs and processes depending on the institution, sorting them, and finally categorizing them accordingly in order to arrive at a *typification* of the institutions in the second murder phase (for theoretical implications, see Kelle and Kluge 2010). Among types such as – to name three immediately obvious cases – the supraregional killing centres (Hadamar, potentially Meseritz-Obrawalde, potentially Großschweidnitz), the mainly regionally operating institutions (see, for example, Sandner 2003, p. 567ff.; Süß 2007) as well as some isolated, rather arbitrary killing initiatives (Faulstich 1998, p. 614), a typology of institutions could be worked out by concentrating on the essentials, "precisely the typical" (Kelle and Kluge 2010, p. 10), which could adequately describe the very complex structure of eugenic action after the supposed euthanasia stop and ultimately make it more tangible.

In addition to the predominantly empirically focused research perspectives listed here, there are also a large number of theoretical follow-up questions to be addressed. The boundaries and limitations are largely open, especially in view of the extensive neglect of the topic in sociology. However, the question of the successful continuation of the operation despite previous formal termination seems to be of particularly great relevance for investigation: The transition from a centrally controlled as well as coordinated action, including an associated authority, to an all in all obviously more decentralized euthanasia campaign, is exceedingly in need of explanation. This change as well as some possible reasons for it have been mentioned in places in the course of this study, but there is no doubt that a much deeper analysis can be made with regard to the question of how such an "overturning" of the once strict guidelines still culminated in a successful continuation of the murder operation. Although the multitude of local studies used here as well as my own explanations can partially trace this transition in the individual empirical cases, a convincing theoretical classification of this phenomenon has so far been lacking.

7.2   Conclusion: Condemnations and Consciousness of Guilt

Q: How do you know the exact dates that these people died?
A: The exact date of death is the date of the day of reception.
Q: How do you know?
A: I knew that they would die on the day that they were received.
Q: How did you know they died, though?
A: Everybody knew that – and I did too. (statement J. Thomas, office staff, Kintner 1948, p. 31)

During its active period, approximately 15,000 lives characterized as "unworthy of life" were exterminated at the LHA Hadamar between 1941 and 1945. It was the only killing facility that was active in both murder phases (Friedlander 1997, p. 264). In the process, more than 10,000 people were gassed, while another 4500–5000 were "euthanized" with pills and syringes. The functionality of the killings was based on several factors: Financial profits, the increasing completion of racial ideological goals in terms of healthy and strong eugenics or ethnicity, as well as (air-)war pragmatic reasons to meet the need for beds or general space in military and general hospitals (Sandner 2003, pp. 606, 638f.). Ultimately, it seems to be above all a combination of these (and sometimes also various other) reasons that have amplified each other in the processes over the years (ibid., p. 653).

Of the euthanasia foot soldiers examined here (see Sect. 1.2), far more people were acquitted than convicted in the German trial (for the following remarks, primarily HHStA/b; also Lilienthal 2006b, p. 288f.; Meusch 2006, p. 314ff.). The guilty verdicts included, among others: Irmgard Huber, accessory to murder in 120 cases, 8 years in prison; Lydia Thomas, accessory to murder in an unspecified number of cases, 5 years in prison; Paul Reuter, accessory to murder in an unspecified number of cases, 4 years and 6 months in prison; Christel Zielke, accessory to murder in at least 25 cases, 3 years and 9 months in prison; Wilhelm Lückoff, accessory to murder in at least eight cases, 3 years and 6 months in prison. A large number of the sentences were vehemently shortened in the course of time. Among others, the defendants Paul Hild, Isabella Weimer, Hubert Gomerski, Maximilian Lindner, Josephine Schirre, and Hannah Bacher were acquitted outright. Meanwhile, the court found the asylum's doctors, Dr. Bodo Gorgaß and Dr. Adolf Wahlmann, guilty of murder in 1000 and 900 cases, respectively, and sentenced them to death. However, both sentences were never actually passed and were transformed into life sentences with the founding of the Federal Republic of Germany instead – which were then in turn gradually reduced, so that Gorgaß was released in 1958 and Wahlmann even in 1953.[3]

At the end of the trial proceedings before the American military court, all seven defendants were found guilty. Alfons Klein, Heinrich Ruoff and Karl Willig were sentenced to death in the course of this. These sentences were all carried out and recorded, including the execution reports that accompanied them (for this, see Kneuker and Steglich 1985, p. 111ff.). Above all, the former senior prison officer Ruoff remained true to his attitude of obedience until the very end:

> I regret that I did not go into the Army at that time. Then I would have been saved great suffering. On the other hand, I would still have my position and my pension; and here I am, now a sick man, an aged man, when I have always been honest. I never did anything wrong. *You can ask all the patients.* That is all. (statement Ruoff, nursing staff, quoted from Kintner 1948, p. 180, emphasis added, DF)

Dr. Adolf Wahlmann received a life sentence, while the defendants Adolf Merkle (35 years), Philipp Blum (30 years) and Irmgard Huber (25 years) were sentenced to comparatively long prison terms.

In regards to the perpetrators' and killers' consciousness of guilt, it should be noted that Lydia Thomas was the only employee who gave an unrestricted admission of guilt (Wettlaufer 1996, p. 310). The judges conceded a lack of consciousness of wrongdoing to the office staff, the technical staff, and another nurse (Meusch 2006, p. 316). Meanwhile, Sister Isabella Weimer, who forced her exit by faking her pregnancy, was the only member of the institution who was able to enforce her release at personal risk (Wettlaufer 1996, p. 312). Weimer had already tried several attempts to escape the institution killings before (statement Weimer, nursing staff, HHStA/a, p. 110).

At the end of these remarks, it would not be too surprising, it seems to me, if interested readers, despite all legal (in-)competence, are somewhat irritated by these final verdicts. At least the author does not feel differently at this point. But perhaps this is also due to the fact that, as already mentioned at the beginning (Sect. 1.2), findings of guilt translated into legal pragmatics are not inevitable determinants of the results of (sociological) thoughts and analyses.

---

[3] Interestingly, Dr. Bodo Gorgaß was living in Bielefeld at the time of the 28.05.1984 (Kneuker and Steglich 1985, p. 53).

Source List

Hessisches Hauptstaatsarchiv Wiesbaden (HHStA), Abt. 461, Nr. 32061, Band 7.

References

Abbott, A. (2004). *Methods of Discovery. Heuristics for the Social Sciences*. New York, London: W. W. Norton & Company.

Adams, G. B. (2011). The Problem of Administrative Evil in a Culture of Technical Rationality. *Public Integrity, 13(3)*, 275–285.

Adams, G. B., & Balfour, D. L. (2009). *Unmasking Administrative Evil*. Armonk & London: M.E. Sharpe.

Adams, G. B., Balfour, D. L., & Reed, G. E. (2006). Abu Gharib, Administrative Evil, and Moral Inversion: The Value of "Putting Cruelty First". *Public Administration Review*, 680–693.

Ahrne, G., & Brunsson, N. (2011). Organization Outside Organizations: The significance of Partial Organization. *Organization, 18(1)*, 83–104.

Ahrne, G., Brunsson, N., & Seidl, D. (2016). Resurrecting Organization by Going Beyond Organizations. *European Management Journal, 34(2)*, 93–101.

Aljets, E., & Hoebel, T. (2017). Prozessuales Erklären. Grundzüge einer primär temporalen Methodologie empirischer Sozialforschung. *Zeitschrift für Soziologie, 46(1)*, 4–21.

Aly, G. (1985a). Der saubere und der schmutzige Fortschritt. In G. Aly, K. F. Masuhr, M. Lehmann, K. H. Roth & U. Schultz (Hrsg.), *Reform und Gewissen. "Euthanasie" im Dienst des Fortschritts. Beiträge zur Nationalsozialistischen Gesundheits- und Sozialpolitik, S. 2* (S. 9–78). Berlin: Rotbuch Verlag.

Aly, G. (1985b). Medizin gegen Unbrauchbare. In G. Aly, A. Ebbinghaus, M. Hamann, F. Pfäfflin & G. Preissler (Hrsg.), *Aussonderung und Tod. Die klinische Hinrichtung der Unbrauchbaren. Beiträge zur Nationalsozialistischen Gesundheits- und Sozialpolitik, S. 1* (S. 9–74). Berlin: Rotbuch Verlag.

Aly, G. (2013). *Die Belasteten. 'Euthanasie' 1939–1945. Eine Gesellschaftsgeschichte.* Bonn: Fischer Verlag GmbH.

Anand, V., Ashforth, B. E., & Joshi, M. (2004). Business as Usual: The Acceptance and Perpetuation of Corruption in Organizations. *Academy of Management Executive, 18(2),* 39–53.

Apelt, M., & Wilkesmann, U. (2015). Einleitung. In M. Apelt & U. Wilkesmann (Hrsg.), *Zur Zukunft der Organisationssoziologie* (S. 9–19). Wiesbaden: Springer VS.

Ashforth, B. E., & Anand, V. (2003). The Normalization of Corruption in Organizations. *Research in Organizational Behavior, 25,* 1–52.

Ashforth, B. E., & Fried, Y. (1988). The Mindlessness of Organizational Behaviors. *Human Relations, 41,* 305–329.

Ashforth, B. E., & Kreiner, G. E. (1999). "How Can You Do It?": Dirty Work and the Challenge of Constructing a Positive Identity. *The Academy of Management Review, 24,* 413–434.

Ashforth, B. E., & Kreiner, G. E. (2002). Normalizing Emotion in Organizations: Making the Extraordinary Seem Ordinary. *Human Resource Management Review, 12,* 215–235.

Ashforth, B. E., Gioia, D. A., Robinson S. L., & Treviño, L. K. (2008). Introduction to Special Topic Forum: Re-Viewing Organizational Corruption. *The Academy of Management Review, 33,* 670–684.

Bajohr, F., & Wildt, M. (2009). Einleitung. In F. Bajohr & M. Wildt (Hrsg.), *Volksgemeinschaft. Neue Forschungen zur Gesellschaft des Nationalsozialismus* (S. 7–23). Frankfurt am Main: Fischer Taschenbuch Verlag

Balcke, J. (2001). *Verantwortungsentlastung durch Organisation. Die "Inspektion der Konzentrationslager und der KZ-Terror".* Tübingen: Edition Diskord.

Bandura, A. (1990). Selective Activation and Disengagement of Moral Control. *Journal of Social Issues, 46(1),* 27–46.

Barnard, C. I. (1938). *The Functions of the Executive.* Cambridge: Harvard University Press.

Baumann, Z. (1992). *Moderne und Ambivalenz. Das Ende der Eindeutigkeit.* Hamburg: Junius.

Becker, M. (2014a). Auf dem Weg zu einer Soziologie des Nationalsozialismus? Zur Entwicklung der soziologischen NS-Forschung seit 1990. In M. Christ & M. Suderland (Hrsg.), *Soziologie und Nationalsozialismus. Positionen, Debatten, Perspektiven* (S. 196–236). Berlin: Suhrkamp.

Becker, M. (2014b). Politik des Beschweigens. Plädoyer für eine historisch-soziologische Rekonstruktion des Verhältnisses der Soziologie zum Nationalsozialismus. *Soziologie, 43(3),* 251–277.

Benedict, S. (2003). Killing While Caring: The Nurses of Hadamar. *Issues in Mental Health Nursing, 24,* 59–79.

Benedict, S., & Kuhla, J. (1999). Nurses' Participation in the Euthanasia Programs of Nazi Germany. *Western Journal of Nursing Research, 21(2),* 246–263.

Bensman, J., & Gerver, I. (1963). Crime and Punishment in the Factory: The Function of Deviancy in Maintaining the Social System. *American Sociological Review, 28(4)*, 588–598.

Benzecry, C. E., Deener A., & Lara-Millián, A. (2020). Archival Work as Qualitative Sociology. *Qualitative Sociology, 43*, 297–303.

Bergmann, J. (1987). *Klatsch. Zur Sozialform der diskreten Indiskretion.* Berlin & New York: Walter de Gruyter.

Bergmann, J. (2013). Gescheiterte Informalität am Beispiel des Korruptionsfalls Siemens. In J. Bergmann, M. Hahn, A. Langhof & G. Wagner (Hrsg.), *Scheitern – Organisations- und wirtschaftssoziologische Analysen* (S. 231–250). Wiesbaden: Springer VS.

Birkenfeld, P., Gabriel, R., & Zeuch, C. (2017). *Die Euthanasie Gedenkstätte Hadamar – Materialsammlung. Eigenständiger Rundgang für Schülerinnen aller Schulformen.* Hadamar: LWV-Hessen.

Borggräfe, H., & Schnitzler, S. (2014). Die Deutsche Gesellschaft für Soziologie und der Nationalsozialismus. Verbandsinterne Transformationen nach 1933 und nach 1945. In M. Christ & M. Suderland (Hrsg.), *Soziologie und Nationalsozialismus. Positionen, Debatten, Perspektiven* (S. 445–479). Berlin: Suhrkamp.

Bosetzky, H. (2019). *Mikropolitik. Netzwerke und Karrieren.* Wiesbaden: Springer VS.

Braun, A. (2016). Zielgerichtete Gewalt zwischen Situation und Identität. School Shootings als identitätsbehauptende Gewaltsituationen. In C. Equit, A. Groenemeyer & H. Schmidt (Hrsg.), *Situationen der Gewalt* (S. 246–261). Weinheim: Beltz Juventa.

Brief, A. P., Buttram, R. T., & Dukerich, J. M. (2001). Collective Corruption in the Corporate World: Toward a Process Model. In M. E. Turner (Hrsg.), *Groups at Work* (S. 471–499). Mahwah: Lawrence Erlbaum Associates.

Broszat, M. (1977): Hitler und die Genesis der "Endlösung". Aus Anlaß der Thesen von David Irving. *Vierteljahreshefte für Zeitgeschichte, 25(4)*, 739–775.

Browning, C. (1989). The Decision Concerning the Final Solution. In: F. Fured (Hrsg.), *Unanswered Questions: Nazi Germany and the Genocide of the Jews* (S. 96–118). New York: Schocken Books.

Brückweh, K. (2009). Dekonstruktion von Prozessakten – Wie ein Strafprozess erzählt werden kann. In J. Finger, S. Keller & A. Wirsching (Hrsg.), *Vom Recht zur Geschichte. Akten aus NS Prozessen als Quellen der Zeitgeschichte* (S. 193–204). Göttingen: Vandenhoeck & Ruprecht.

Bryant, M. S. (2005). *Confronting the "Good Death". Nazi Euthanasia on Trial, 1945–1953.* Colorado: University Press of Colorado.

Burlon, M. (2009). *Die "Euthanasie" an Kindern während des Nationalsozialismus in den zwei Hamburger Kinderfachabteilungen.* Hamburg: Universität Hamburg.

Campbell, J.-L., & Göritz, A. S. (2014). Culture Corrupts! A Qualitative Study of Organizational Culture in Corrupt Organizations. *Journal of Business Ethics, 120*, 291–311.

Card, R. F. (2005). Individual Responsibility within Organizational Contexts. *Journal of Business Ethics, 62*, 397–405.

Christ, M. (2011). Die Soziologie und das 'Dritte Reich'. Weshalb Holocaust und Nationalsozialismus in der Soziologie ein Schattendasein führen. *Soziologie, 40(4)*, 407–431.

Christ, M. (2014). Gewalt in der Moderne. Holocaust und Nationalsozialismus in der soziologischen Gewaltforschung. In M. Christ & M. Suderland (Hrsg.), *Soziologie und Nationalsozialismus. Positionen, Debatten, Perspektiven* (S. 332–364). Berlin: Suhrkamp.

Christ, M., & Suderland, M. (2014). Der Nationalsozialismus – (k)ein Thema für die Soziologie? In M. Christ & M. Suderland (Hrsg.), Soziologie und Nationalsozialismus. Positionen, Debatten, Perspektiven (S. 13–30). Berlin: Suhrkamp.

Chroust, P., Groß, H., Hamann M., & Sörensen, J. (1989). "Soll nach Hadamar überführt werden". Den Opfern der Euthanasiemorde 1939 bis 1945. Gedenkausstellung in Hadamar, Katalog. Frankfurt am Main: Mabuse.

Cicourel, A. V. (1974). Methode und Messung in der Soziologie. Frankfurt am Main: Suhrkamp.

Collins, R. (2009). The Micro-Sociology of Violence. The British Journal of Sociology, 60(3), 566–576.

Collins, R. (2011). Dynamik der Gewalt. Eine mikrosoziologische Theorie. Hamburg: Hamburger Edition.

Culjak, A. (2015). Organisation und Devianz. Eine empirische Fallrekonstruktion der Havarie der Costa Concordia. Wiesbaden: Springer VS.

Dahrendorf, R. (1989). Soziologie und Nationalsozialismus. In H.-J. Hoffmann-Nowotny (Hrsg.), Kultur und Gesellschaft: gemeinsamer Kongreß der Deutschen, der Österreichischen und der Schweizerischen Gesellschaft für Soziologie (S. 669–675). Zürich: Seismo Verlag.

Daum, M. (1996). Arbeit und Zwang, das Leben der Hadamarer Patienten im Schatten des Todes. In D. Roer & D. Henkel (Hrsg.), Psychiatrie im Faschismus. Die Anstalt Hadamar 1933–1945 (S. 173–213). Bonn: Psychiatrie-Verlag.

Debus, D., Kalkowsky, B., & Schmidt-von Blittersdorff, H. (1996). Neuere Überlegungen zur Vorbereitung und Organisation der Verbrechen der Psychiatrie in der NS-Zeit. In D. Roer & D. Henkel (Hrsg.), Psychiatrie im Faschismus. Die Anstalt Hadamar 1933–1945 (S. 38–57). Bonn: Psychiatrie-Verlag.

Ebbinghaus, A. (2008). Mediziner vor Gericht. In K.-D. Henke (Hrsg.), Tödliche Medizin im Nationalsozialismus. Von der Rassenhygiene zum Massenmord (S. 203–224). Köln: Böhlau Verlag.

Eckart, W. U. (2011). Universitäten, Studierende, Medizinische Fakultäten. In R. Jütte (Hrsg.), Medizin und Nationalsozialismus. Bilanz und Perspektiven der Forschung (S. 106–123). Göttingen: Wallstein Verlag.

Ermann, M. D., & Lundman, R. J. (1978). Deviant Acts by Complex Organizations: Deviance and Social Control at the Organizational Level of Analysis. The Sociological Quarterly, 19(1), 55–67.

Falleti, T. G., & Mahoney, J. (2015). The Comparative Sequential Method. In J. Mahoney & K. Thelen (Hrsg.), Advances in Comparative-Historical Analysis (S. 211–239). New York: Cambridge University Press.

Faulstich, H. (1998). Hungersterben in der Psychiatrie 1914–1949. Mit einer Topographie der NS-Psychiatrie. Freiburg im Breisgau: Lambertus-Verlag.

Finger, J., & Keller, S. (2009). Täter und Opfer – Gedanken zu Quellenkritik und Aussagekontext. In J. Finger, S. Keller & A. Wirsching (Hrsg.), Vom Recht zur Geschichte. Akten aus NS-Prozessen als Quellen der Zeitgeschichte (S. 114–131). Göttingen: Vandenhoeck & Ruprecht.

Finger, J., Keller, S., & Wirsching, A. (2009). Einleitung. In J. Finger, S. Keller & A. Wirsching (Hrsg.), Vom Recht zur Geschichte. Akten aus NS-Prozessen als Quellen der Zeitgeschichte (S. 9–24). Göttingen: Vandenhoeck & Ruprecht.

Firkus, D. (2017). *Eine genuine Soziologie der Gewalt? Empirisch gestützte Überlegungen zur Erklärungskraft der Gewalttheorie Randall Collins'*. Bielefeld: Universität Bielefeld.

Firkus, D. (2021). Harzburg und die Suche nach Kontinuität. Rezension zu "Gehorsam macht frei. Eine kurze Geschichte des Managements – von Hitler bis heute" von Johann Chapoutot. https://www.soziopolis.de/harzburg-und-die-suche-nach-kontinuitaet.html. Accessed on: 21.05.2021.

Flyvbjerg, B. (2006). Five Misunderstandings About Case-Study Research. *Qualitative Inquiry, 12(2)*, 219–245.

Friedlander, H. (1997). *Der Weg zum NS-Genozid. Von der Euthanasie zur Endlösung.* Berlin: Berlin Verlag.

Friedrich, S. (2012). *Soziologie des Genozids. Grenzen und Möglichkeiten einer Forschungsperspektive.* München: Wilhelm Fink Verlag.

George, U. (2006). "Erholte sich nicht mehr. Heute exitus an Marasmus senilis". Die Opfer der Jahre 1942–1945 in Hadamar. In U. George, G. Lilienthal, V. Roelcke, P. Sandner & C. Vanja (Hrsg.), *Hadamar. Heilstätte – Tötungsanstalt – Therapiezentrum* (S. 234–258). Marburg: Jonas Verlag

Gerth, H., & Mills, C. W. (1973). Motivvokabulare. In H. Steinert (Hrsg.), *Symbolische Interaktion. Arbeiten zu einer reflexiven Soziologie* (S. 156–161). Stuttgart: Klett Verlag.

Gioia, D. A. (1992). Pinto Fires and Personal Ethics: A Script Analysis of Missed Opportunities. *Journal of Business Ethics, 11*, 379–389.

Gioia, D. A., & Poole, P. P. (1984). Scripts in Organizational Behavior. *Academy of Management Review, 9(3)*, 449–459.

Greil, A. L., & Rudy, D. R. (1984). Social Cocoons: Encapsulation and Identity Transformation Organizations. *Sociological Inquiry, 54*, 260–278.

Gruber, A. (2015). "…zunächst wurde nach Freiwilligen gesucht." Soziologische Erklärungsansätze zur freiwilligen Beteiligung von Ordnungspolizisten an der "Endlösung". In A. Gruber & S. Kühl (Hrsg.), *Soziologische Analysen des Holocaust* (S. 29–54). Wiesbaden: Springer VS.

Gruber, A. (2017). Warum lässt man sich führen? Elementare, formale und informale Führung. In C. Barthel & D. Heidemann (Hrsg.), *Führung in der Polizei. Bausteine für ein soziologisch informiertes Führungsverständnis* (S. 217–244). Wiesbaden: Springer VS.

Gruber, A., & Kühl, S. (2015). Autoritätsakzeptanz und Folgebereitschaft in Organisationen. Zur Beteiligung der Mitglieder des Reserve-Polizeibataillons 101 am Holocaust. In A. Gruber & S. Kühl (Hrsg.), *Soziologische Analysen des Holocaust* (S. 7–28). Wiesbaden: Springer VS.

Hartz, R. (2020). "Organisationen und X" – Neuere Literatur zur Organisationssoziologie und -forschung. *Soziologische Revue, 43(2)*, 185–210.

Hauffe, T. (2013). *Hier ist kein Warum. Willkür in den nationalsozialistischen Konzentrationslagern – eine soziologische Analyse.* Unveröffentlichte Diplomarbeit. Bielefeld: Universität Bielefeld.

Herrmann, D. (1987). Die Konstruktion von Realität in Justizakten. *Zeitschrift für Soziologie, 16(1)*, 44–55.

Hilberg, R. (1989). The Bureaucracy of Annihilation. In F. Furet (Hrsg.), *Unanswered Questions: Nazi Germany and the Genocide of the Jews* (S. 119–133). New York: Schocken Books.

Hinz-Wessels, A. (2002). Das Schicksal jüdischer Patienten in brandenburgischen Heil- und Pflegeanstalten im Nationalsozialismus. In K. Hübener (Hrsg.), *Brandenburgische Heil- und Pflegeanstalten in der NS-Zeit* (S. 259–286). Berlin: be.bra Verlag.

Hinz-Wessels, A., Fuchs, P., Hohendorf, G., & Rotzoll, M. (2005). Zur bürokratischen Abwicklung eines Massenmordes. Die "Euthanasie"-Aktion im Spiegel neuer Dokumente. *Vierteljahreshefte für Zeitgeschichte, 53(1)*, 79–107.

Hirschinger, F. (2001). *"Zur Ausmerzung freigegeben". Halle und die Landesheilanstalt Altscherbitz 1933–1945*. Köln, Weimer & Wien: Böhlau Verlag.

Hoebel, T. (2014). Organisierte Plötzlichkeit. Eine prozesssoziologische Erklärung antisymmetrischer Gewaltsituationen. *Zeitschrift für Soziologie, 43(6)*, 441–457.

Hoebel, T. (2018). Normalisierung des Absurden? Das "Simon-und-Garfinkel-Prinzip" und die kommunikative Validierung von Nonsens. In E. Heitzer & S. Schultze (Hrsg.), *Chimära mensura? Die Human-Animal Studies zwischen Schäferhund-Science-Hoax, kritischer Geschichtswissenschaft und akademischem Trendsurfing* (S. 176–190). Berlin: Vergangenheitsverlag.

Hoffmann, U. (2010). Normale Leute? Kollektivbiografische Anmerkungen zu den Tätern der NS-"Euthanasie". In M. Rotzoll, G. Hohendorf, P. Fuchs, P. Richter, C. Mundt & W. U. Eckart (Hrsg.), *Die nationalsozialistische "Euthanasie"-Aktion "T4" und ihre Opfer. Geschichte und ethische Konsequenzen für die Gegenwart* (S. 252–258). Paderborn, München, Wien & Zürich: Ferdinand Schöningh.

Höhn, R. (1934). *Das Wissen um die Gemeinschaft: Vom Wesen der Gemeinschaft*. Berlin: Carl Heymanns Verlag.

Höhn, R. (1969). *Führungsbrevier der Wirtschaft*. Bad Harzburg: Verlag für Wissenschaft, Wirtschaft und Technik.

Jütte, R. (2011). Krankenpflege. In R. Jütte (Hrsg.), *Medizin und Nationalsozialismus. Bilanz und Perspektiven der Forschung* (S. 94–105). Göttingen: Wallstein Verlag.

Kaiser, J.-C., Nowak, K., & Schwartz, M. (1992). *Eugenik. Sterilisation. Euthanasie. Politische Biologie in Deutschland 1895–1945. Eine Dokumentation*. Berlin: Buchverlag Union.

Kaptein, M., & van Helvoort, M. (2018). A Model of Neutralization Techniques. *Deviant Behavior, 40(10)*, 1–26.

Katz, F. E. (1982). Implementation of the Holocaust: The Behavior of Nazi Officials. *Comparative Studies in Society and History, 24*, 510–529.

Katz, F. E. (1993). *Ordinary People and Extraordinary Evil. A Report on the Beguilings of Evil*. Albany: State University of New York Press.

Katz, J. (2016). A Theory of Intimate Massacres: Steps Toward a Causal Explanation. *Theoretical Criminology, 20*, 277–296.

Kaufmann, H., & Schulmeyer, K. (1996). Die polnischen und sowjetischen Zwangsarbeiter in Hadamar. In D. Roer & D. Henkel (Hrsg.), *Psychiatrie im Faschismus. Die Anstalt Hadamar 1933–1945* (S. 256–282). Bonn: Psychiatrie-Verlag.

Kelle, U., & Kluge, S. (2010). *Vom Einzelfall zum Typus. Fallvergleich und Fallkontrastierung in der qualitativen Sozialforschung*. Wiesbaden: VS Verlag.

Kepplinger, B. (2008). Die Tötungsanstalt Hartheim 1940–1945. In B. Kepplinger, G. Marckhgott & H. Reese (Hrsg.), *Tötungsanstalt Hartheim* (S. 63–116). Linz: Oberösterreichisches Landesarchiv.

Keßelring, A. (2018). Die historische Analyse paramilitärischer Verbände als Herausforderung für die Neueste Militärgeschichte am Beispiel der Kommandoverantwortung im zerfallenden Jugoslawien. *Militärgeschichtliche Zeitschrift, 77(2)*, 415–457.

Kieserling, A. (2012). Funktionen und Folgen formaler Organisation (1964). In O. Jahraus, A. Nassehi, M. Grizelj, I. Saake & C. Kirchmeier (Hrsg.), *Luhmann-Handbuch: Leben-Werk-Wirkung* (S. 129–135). Stuttgart, Weimar: Metzler.

Kintner, E. W. (1948). *Trial of Alfons Klein, Adolf Wahlmann, Heinrich Ruoff, Karl Willig, Adolf Merkle, Irmgard Huber and Philipp Blum. The Hadamar Trial.* London, Edinburgh, Glasgow: William Hodge and Company.

Klatetzki, T. (2015). "Hang em high". Der Lynchmob als temporäre Organisation. In A. T. Paul & B. Schwalb (Hrsg.), *Gewaltmassen. Über Eigendynamik und Selbstorganisation kollektiver Gewalt* (S. 147–172). Hamburg: Hamburger Edition.

Klee, E. (1983). *"Euthanasie" im NS-Staat. Die "Vernichtung lebensunwerten Lebens".* Frankfurt am Main: S. Fischer Verlag.

Klee, E. (1986). *Dokumente zur Euthanasie.* Frankfurt am Main: Fischer Taschenbuch Verlag.

Kneuker, G., & Steglich, W. (1985). *Begegnungen mit der Euthanasie in Hadamar.* Rehburg-Loccum: Psychiatrie-Verlag.

Koessler, M. (1953). Euthanasia in the Hadamar Sanatorium and International Law. *Journal of Criminal Law and Criminology, 43(6)*, 735–755.

Kreiner, G. E., Ashforth, B. E., & Sluss, D. M. (2006). Identity Dynamics in Occupational Dirty Work: Integrating Social Identity and System Justification Perspectives. *Organization Science, 17(5)*, 619–636.

Kühl, S. (1994). *The Nazi Connection. Eugeneics, American Racism, and German National Socialism.* New York, Oxford: Oxford University Press.

Kühl, S. (2005). Ganz normale Organisationen. Organisationssoziologische Interpretationen simulierter Brutalitäten. *Zeitschrift für Soziologie, 34*, 90–111.

Kühl, S. (2007a). Formalität, Informalität und Illegalität in der Organisationsberatung. Systemtheoretische Analyse eines Beratungsprozesses. *Soziale Welt, 58*, 269–291.

Kühl, S. (2007b). Wie normal sind die ganz normalen Organisationen? Zur Interpretation des Deportations-, Milgram-, Stanford-Prison und Soda-Cracker-Experiments. *Working Paper 2/2007.* Bielefeld: Universität Bielefeld.

Kühl, S. (2007c). Willkommen im Club. Zur Diskussion über die Organisationshaftigkeit des Deportations-, Soda-Cracker-, Stanford-Prison- und Milgram-Experiments. *Zeitschrift für Soziologie, 36*, 313–319.

Kühl, S. (2011). *Organisationen. Eine sehr kurze Einführung.* Wiesbaden: Springer VS.

Kühl, S. (2013a). Ein letzter kläglicher Versuch der Verdrängung. Zur Diskussion über den Ort des Nationalsozialismus in der Soziologie. *Working Paper 5/2013.* Bielefeld: Universität Bielefeld.

Kühl, S. (2013b). Im Prinzip ganz einfach. Zur Klärung des Verhältnisses der Soziologie zum Nationalsozialismus. *Working Paper 6/2013.* Bielefeld: Universität Bielefeld.

Kühl, S. (2013c). Zur Rolle der "ganz normalen Organisationen" im Holocaust. Vorüberlegungen zu einem Buchprojekt. *Working Paper 4/2013.* Bielefeld: Universität Bielefeld.

Kühl, S. (2014a). *Ganz normale Organisationen. Zur Soziologie des Holocaust.* Berlin: Suhrkamp Verlag.

Kühl, S. (2014b). Gruppen, Organisationen, Familien und Bewegungen. Zur Soziologie mitgliedschaftsbasierter Systeme zwischen Interaktion und Gesellschaft. *Zeitschrift für Soziologie, Sonderheft "Interaktion, Organisation und Gesellschaft"*, 65–85.

Kühl, S. (2015). Gesellschaft der Organisationen, organisierte Gesellschaft, Organisationsgesellschaft. Zu den Grenzen einer an Organisationen ansetzenden Zeitdiagnose. In M. Apelt & U. Wilkesmann (Hrsg.), *Zur Zukunft der Organisationssoziologie* (S. 73–91). Wiesbaden: Springer VS.

Kühl, S. (2017a). Die Holocaustforschung beforscht sich selbst. Soziologische Perspektiven auf die Probleme der Zeitgeschichtsforschung. *Working Paper 16/2017*. Bielefeld: Universität Bielefeld.

Kühl, S. (2017b). Zur Erosion von Kameradschaft. Informale Normen in staatlichen Gewaltorganisationen. *Working Paper 15/2017*. Bielefeld: Universität Bielefeld.

Kühl, S. (2018/2019). Ganz normale Organisationen? Zur Kritik eines systemtheoretischen Zugangs in der Holocaustforschung. *Mittelweg, 36(6)*, 104–127.

Kühl, S. (2019a). Familien und Organisationen: Gemeinsamkeiten, Unterschiede und Verknüpfungen. In H. Kleve & T. Köllner (Hrsg.), *Soziologie der Unternehmerfamilie. Grundlagen, Entwicklungslinien, Perspektiven* (S. 99–113). Wiesbaden: Springer VS.

Kühl, S. (2019b). Von der notwendigen Unterscheidung von Gruppe und Organisation. *Working Paper 9/2019*. Bielefeld: Universität Bielefeld.

Kühl, S. (2020a). *Brauchbare Illegalität. Vom Nutzen des Regelbruchs in Organisationen.* Frankfurt & New York: Campus Verlag.

Kühl, S. (2020b). Zwischen Präzision und Anonymisierung. Wie weit muss man bei der Verfälschung wissenschaftlicher Daten gehen? *Soziologie, 49(1)*, 62–71.

Lehnstaedt, S. (2017). *Der Kern des Holocaust. Belzec, Sobibór, Treblinka und die Aktion Reinhardt.* München: C. H. Beck.

Lelle, N. (2018). Was bedeutet Fortleben der Vergangenheit? "Deutsche Arbeit" in der frühen Nachkriegszeit. In F. Axster & N. Lelle (Hrsg.), *"Deutsche Arbeit". Kritische Perspektiven auf ein ideologisches Selbstbild* (S. 54–75). Wallstein: Wallstein Verlag.

Lewandowski, S. (2019). Die Praxen der Amateurpornographie. www.Svenlewandowski. de/108201.html. Accessed on: 02.10.2020.

Lifton, R. J. (1988). *Ärzte im Dritten Reich.* Stuttgart: Klett-Cotta.

Lilienthal, G. (2006a). Gaskammer und Überdosis. Die Landesheilanstalt Hadamar als Mordzentrum (1941–1945). In U. George, G. Lilienthal, V. Roelcke, P. Sandner & C. Vanja (Hrsg.), *Hadamar. Heilstätte – Tötungsanstalt – Therapiezentrum* (S. 156–175). Marburg: Jonas Verlag.

Lilienthal, G. (2006b). Personal einer Tötungsanstalt. Acht biographische Skizzen. In U. George, G. Lilienthal, V. Roelcke, P. Sandner & C. Vanja (Hrsg.), *Hadamar. Heilstätte – Tötungsanstalt – Therapiezentrum* (S. 267–292). Marburg: Jonas Verlag.

Lilienthal, G. (2009). Jüdische Patienten als Opfer der NS-"Euthansie"-Verbrechen. *Magazin für jüdisches Leben in Forschung und Bildung, 5*, 1–16.

Lilienthal, G. (2010). Von der "zentralen" zur "kooperativen Euthanasie". Die Tötungsanstalt Hadamar und die "T4" (1942–1945). In M. Rotzoll, G. Hohendorf, P. Fuchs, P. Richter, C. Mundt & W. U. Eckart (Hrsg.), *Die nationalsozialistische "Euthanasie"-Aktion "T4" und ihre Opfer. Geschichte und ethische Konsequenzen für die Gegenwart* (S. 100–110). Paderborn, München, Wien & Zürich: Ferdinand Schöningh.

Luft, A. (2020). How Do you Repair a Broken World? Conflict(ing) Archives after the Holocaust. *Qualitative Sociology, 43*, 317–343.

Luhmann, N. (1983). *Legitimation durch Verfahren.* Frankfurt am Main: Suhrkamp Verlag.
Luhmann, N. (1987). *Rechtssoziologie.* Opladen: Westdeutscher Verlag.
Luhmann, N. (1995). *Funktionen und Folgen formaler Organisationen.* Berlin: Duncker & Humblot.
Luhmann, N. (2005). Interaktion, Organisation, Gesellschaft. Anwendungen der Systemtheorie. In N. Luhmann (Hrsg.), *Soziologische Aufklärung 2. Aufsätze zur Theorie der Gesellschaft* (S. 9–24). Wiesbaden: Springer VS.
Luhmann, N. (2018a). Der neue Chef. In E. Lukas & V. Tacke (Hrsg.), *Schriften zur Organisation 1. Die Wirklichkeit der Organisation* (S. 275–291). Wiesbaden: Springer VS.
Luhmann, N. (2018b). Formale Struktur und richtiges Handeln. In E. Lukas & V. Tacke (Hrsg.), *Schriften zur Organisation 1. Die Wirklichkeit der Organisation* (S. 135–151). Wiesbaden: Springer VS.
Luhmann, N. (2018c). Gesellschaftliche Organisation. In E. Lukas & V. Tacke (Hrsg.), *Schriften zur Organisation 1. Die Wirklichkeit der Organisation* (S. 385–413). Wiesbaden: Springer VS.
Luhmann, N. (2018d). Unterwachung. Oder die Kunst, Vorgesetzte zu lenken. In E. Lukas & V. Tacke (Hrsg.), *Schriften zur Organisation 1. Die Wirklichkeit der Organisation* (S. 415–424). Wiesbaden: Springer VS.
Mann, M. (2000). Were the Perpetrators of Genocide "Ordinary Men" or "Real Nazis?" Results From Fifteen Hundred Biographies. *Holocaust and Genocide Studies, 14(3),* 331–366.
Maruna, S., & Copes, H. (2005). What Have We Learned From Five Decades of Neutralization Research? *Crimes and Justice, 32,* 221–320.
Masuch, M. (1985). Vicious Circles in Organizations. *Administrative Science Quarterly, 30,* 14–33.
McCabe, D., & Hamilton, L. (2015). The Kill Programme: An Ethnographic Study of 'Dirty Work' in a Slaughterhouse. *New Technology, Work and Employment, 30(2),* 95–108.
Meusch, M. (2006). Die strafrechtliche Verfolgung der Hadamarer "Euthanasie"-Morde. In U. George, G. Lilienthal, V. Roelcke, P. Sandner & C. Vanja (Hrsg.), *Hadamar. Heilstätte – Tötungsanstalt – Therapiezentrum* (S. 305–326). Marburg: Jonas Verlag.
Mills, C. W. (1940). Situated Actions and Vocabularies of Motive. *American Sociological Review, 5,* 904– 913.
Mitscherlich, A., & Mielke, F. (1995). *Medizin ohne Menschlichkeit. Dokumente des Nürnberger Ärzteprozesses.* Frankfurt am Main: Fischer Taschenbuch Verlag.
Müthel, M. (2017). Pro-organisationales illegales Verhalten. Wie und warum gute Mitarbeiter dem Unternehmen schaden. *Zeitschrift Führung+Organisation, 86,* 31–36.
Nassauer, A. (2016). Theoretische Überlegungen zur Entstehung von Gewalt in Protesten: Eine situative mechanismische Erklärung. *Berliner Journal für Soziologie, 25,* 491–518.
Neidhardt, F. (1979). Das innere System sozialer Gruppen. *Kölner Zeitschrift für Soziologie und Sozialpsychologie, 31(4),* 639–660.
Neidhardt, F. (1983). Themen und Thesen zur Gruppensoziologie. *Kölner Zeitschrift für Soziologie und Sozialpsychologie, 25,* 12–34.
Osrecki, F. (2015). Kritischer Funktionalismus: Über die Grenzen und Möglichkeiten einer kritischen Systemtheorie. *Soziale Systeme, 20,* 1–30.
Paul, A. T. & Schwalb, B. (2012). Kriminelle Organisationen. In M. Apelt & V. Tacke (Hrsg.), *Handbuch Organisationstypen* (S. 327–344). Wiesbaden: Springer VS.

Perrow, C. (2009). Foreword to the Revisited Edition. In G. B. Adams & D. L. Balfour, *Unmasking Administrative Evil* (S. xxvii–xxxix). Armonk & London: M.E. Sharpe.

Pierson, P. (2003). Big, Slow-Moving and … Invisible. Macrosocial Processes in the Study of Comparative Politics. In J. Mahoney & D. Rueschemeyer (Hrsg.), *Comparative Historical Analysis in the Social Sciences* (S. 177–207). Cambridge: University Press.

Pinto, J., Leana, C. R., & Pil, F. K. (2008). Corrupt Organizations or Organizations of Corrupt Individuals? Two Types of Organization-Level Corruption. *Academy of Management Review, 33,* 685–709.

Pütz, O., & Meier zu Verl, C. (2014). Grillen als soziale Praxis. Eine ethnomethodologische Rekonstruktion. In S. Szabo & H. Köpper (Hrsg.), *BBQ. Grillen – eine Wissenschaft für sich: Antworten der Forschung auf ein Massenphänomen* (S. 163–176). Marburg: Tectum Verlag.

Reed, G. E. (2012). Leading Questions: Leadership, Ethics, and Administrative Evil. *Leadership, 8(2),* 187–198.

Roer, D. (1992). Psychiatrie in Deutschland 1933–1945: ihr Beitrag zur "Endlösung der Sozialen Frage", am Beispiel der Heilanstalt Uchtspringe. *Psychologie und Gesellschaftskritik, 16,* 15–37.

Roer, D., & Henkel, D. (1996a). In D. Roer & D. Henkel (Hrsg.), *Psychiatrie im Faschismus. Die Anstalt Hadamar 1933–1945* (S. 7–12). Bonn: Psychiatrie-Verlag.

Roer, D., & Henkel, D. (1996b). Funktion bürgerlicher Psychiatrie und ihre besondere Form im Faschismus. In D. Roer & D. Henkel (Hrsg.), *Psychiatrie im Faschismus. Die Anstalt Hadamar 1933–1945* (S. 13–37). Bonn: Psychiatrie-Verlag.

Sandberg, J., & Alvesson, M. (2011). Ways of Constructing Research Questions: Gap-Spotting or Problematization? *Organization, 18(1),* 23–44.

Sandkühler, T. (2020). *Das Fußvolk der "Endlösung". Nichtdeutsche Täter und die europäische Dimension des Völkermords.* Darmstadt: wbgAcademic.

Sandner, P. (1999). Die "Euthanasie"-Akten im Bundesarchiv. Zur Geschichte eines lange verschollenen Bestandes *Vierteljahreshefte für Zeitgeschichte, 47(3),* 385–400.

Sandner, P. (2003). *Verwaltung des Krankenmordes. Der Bezirksverband Nassau im Nationalsozialismus.* Harland, Wirth: Psychosozial-Verlag.

Sandner, P. (2006). Die Landesheilanstalt Hadamar 1933–1945 als Einrichtung des Bezirksverbandes Nassau (Wiesbaden). In U. George, G. Lilienthal, V. Roelcke, P. Sandner & C. Vanja (Hrsg.), *Hadamar. Heilstätte – Tötungsanstalt – Therapiezentrum* (S. 136–155). Marburg: Jonas Verlag.

Schimank, U. (2015). Zu viele lose Fäden – und ein paar Schlingen um den Hals. Randnotizen zum Wissensstand der Organisationssoziologie. In M. Apelt & U. Wilkesmann (Hrsg.), *Zur Zukunft der Organisationssoziologie* (S. 293–306). Wiesbaden: Springer.

Schmidt, M., Kuhlmann, R., & von Cranach, M. (2012). Heil- und Pflegeanstalt Kaufbeuren. In M. von Cranach & H.-L. Siemen (Hrsg.), *Psychiatrie im Nationalsozialismus. Die Bayerischen Heil- und Pflegeanstalten zwischen 1933 und 1945* (S. 265–325). München: Oldenbourg Verlag.

Schmidt-von Blittersdorff, H., Debus, D., & Kalkowsky, B. (1996). Die Geschichte der Anstalt Hadamar von 1933 bis 1945 und ihre Funktion im Rahmen von T4. In D. Roer & D. Henkel (Hrsg.), *Psychiatrie im Faschismus. Die Anstalt Hadamar 1933–1945* (S. 58–120). Bonn: Psychiatrie-Verlag.

Schmuhl, H.-W. (2008). Die biopolitische Entwicklungsdiktatur des Nationalsozialismus und der "Reichsgesundheitsführer" Leonardo Conti. In K.-D. Henke (Hrsg.), *Tödliche*

Medizin im Nationalsozialismus. Von der Rassenhygiene zum Massenmord (S. 101–117). Köln: Böhlau Verlag.

Schmuhl, H.-W. (2011a). Eugenik und Rassenanthropologie. In R. Jütte (Hrsg.), *Medizin und Nationalsozialismus. Bilanz und Perspektiven der Forschung* (S. 24–38). Göttingen: Wallstein Verlag.

Schmuhl, H.-W. (2011b). Zwangssterilisation. In R. Jütte (Hrsg.), *Medizin und Nationalsozialismus. Bilanz und Perspektiven der Forschung* (S. 201–213). Göttingen: Wallstein Verlag.

Schmuhl, H.-W. (2011c). "Euthanasie" und Krankenmord. In R. Jütte (Hrsg.), *Medizin und Nationalsozialismus. Bilanz und Perspektiven der Forschung* (S. 214–255). Göttingen: Wallstein Verlag.

Soeffner, H.-G. (2014). Arbeit an Entlastungsmythen. Geleitwort. In M. Christ & M. Suderland (Hrsg.), *Soziologie und Nationalsozialismus. Positionen, Debatten, Perspektiven* (S. 9–12). Berlin: Suhrkamp.

Stöckle, T. (2010). Die Reaktion der Angehörigen und der Bevölkerung auf die "Aktion T4". In M. Rotzoll, G. Hohendorf, P. Fuchs, P. Richter, C. Mundt & W. U. Eckart (Hrsg.), *Die nationalsozialistische "Euthanasie"-Aktion "T4" und ihre Opfer. Geschichte und ethische Konsequenzen für die Gegenwart* (S. 118–124). Paderborn, München, Wien & Zürich: Ferdinand Schöningh.

Suderland, M. (2014). "Das Konzentrationslager als giftigste Beule des Terrors". Soziologische Perspektive auf die nationalsozialistischen Zwangslager. In M. Christ & M. Suderland (Hrsg.), *Soziologie und Nationalsozialismus. Positionen, Debatten, Perspektiven* (S. 365–405). Berlin: Suhrkamp.

Süß, W. (2003). *Der "Volkskörper" im Krieg. Gesundheitspolitik, Gesundheitsverhältnisse und Krankenmord im nationalsozialistischen Deutschland 1939–1945*. München: Oldenbourg Verlag.

Süß, W. (2007). Dezentralisierter Krankenmord. Zum Verhältnis von Zentralgewalt und Regionalgewalt in der "Euthanasie" seit 1942. In J. John, H. Möller & T. Schaarschmidt (Hrsg.), *Die NS-Gaue. Regionale Mittelinstanzen im zentralistischen "Führerstaat"?* (S. 123–135). Oldenbourg: De Gruyter.

Sykes, G. M., & Matza, D. (1957). Techniques of Neutralization: A Theory of Delinquency. *American Sociological Review, 22(6)*, 664–670.

Tacke, V. (2010). Organisationssoziologie. In G. Kneer & M. Schroer (Hrsg.), *Handbuch Spezielle Soziologien* (S. 341–359). Wiesbaden: VS Verlag.

Tacke, V. (2015). Perspektiven der Organisationssoziologie. Ein Essay über Risiken und Nebenwirkungen des Erfolgs. In M. Apelt & U. Wilkesmann (Hrsg.), *Zur Zukunft der Organisationssoziologie* (S. 273–292). Wiesbaden: Springer VS.

Tacke, V., & Drepper, T. (2018). *Soziologie der Organisation*. Wiesbaden: Springer VS.

Weißmann, M. (2015). Organisierte Entmenschlichung. Zur Produktion, Funktion und Ersetzbarkeit sozialer und psychischer Dehumanisierung in Genoziden. In A. Gruber & S. Kühl (Hrsg.), *Soziologische Analysen des Holocaust* (S. 79–128). Wiesbaden: Springer VS.

Welzer, H. (2005). *Täter. Wie aus ganz normalen Menschen Massenmörder werden*. Frankfurt am Main: Fischer Verlag.

Werner, W. F. (1991). Die Rheinprovinz und die Tötungsanstalt Hadamar. In C. Vanja & M. Vogt (Hrsg.), *Euthanasie in Hadamar. Die nationalsozialistische Vernichtungspoli-*

tik in hessischen Anstalten. Begleitband (S. 135–143). Kassel: Landeswohlfahrtsverband Hessen.

Wettlaufer, A. (1996). Die Beteiligung von Schwestern und Pflegern an den Morden in Hadamar. In D. Roer & D. Henkel (Hrsg.), *Psychiatrie im Faschismus. Die Anstalt Hadamar 1933–1945* (S. 283–330). Bonn: Psychiatrie-Verlag.

Wildt, M. (2011). Der Fall Reinhard Höhn. Vom Reichssicherheitshauptamt zur Harzburger Akademie. In A. Gallus & A. Schildt (Hrsg.), *Rückblickend in die Zukunft. Politische Öffentlichkeit und intellektuelle Positionen in Deutschland um 1950 und um 1930* (S. 254–271). Göttingen: Wallstein Verlag.

Winter, B. (1991). Hadamar als T4-Anstalt 1941–1945. In C. Vanja & M. Vogt (Hrsg.), *Euthanasie in Hadamar. Die nationalsozialistische Vernichtungspolitik in hessischen Anstalten. Begleitband* (S. 91–104). Kassel: Landeswohlfahrtsverband Hessen.

Zimbardo, P. G. (2009). Foreword to the Third Edition. In G. B. Adams & D. L. Balfour, *Unmasking Administrative Evil* (S. ix–xvi). Armonk & London: M.E. Sharpe.

The manufacturer's authorised representative in the EU is Springer
Nature Customer Service Centre GmbH, Europaplatz 3, 69115 Heidelberg,
Germany. If you have any concerns regarding our products, please
contact ProductSafety@springernature.com

Printed and bound by CPI Group (UK) Ltd, Croydon, CR0 4YY
28/04/2026
02098539-0003